From Belly Fat to Belly **FLAT**

How Your Hormones Are Adding
Inches to Your Waistline and
Subtracting Years from Your Life

The MEDICALLY PROVEN Way
to RESHAPE YOUR BODY

C.W. Randolph, Jr., M.D.
author of *From Hormone Hell to Hormone Well*
and **Genie James**

Health Communications, Inc.
Deerfield Beach, Florida

www.hcibooks.com

Library of Congress Cataloging-in-Publication Data

Randolph, C.W.
    From belly fat to belly flat / C.W. Randolph and Genie James.
      p. cm.
    ISBN-13: 978-0-7573-0678-5 (trade paper)
    ISBN-10: 0-7573-0678-0 (trade paper)
      1. Weight loss—Endocrine aspects.   2. Estrogen—Physiological effect.
    I. James, Genie.   II. Title.
    RM222.2.R358 2008
    613.2'5—dc22

                                    2007035748

Publisher: Health Communications, Inc.
               3201 S.W. 15th Street
               Deerfield Beach, FL 33442-8190

R-04-08

Cover design by Larissa Hise Henoch
Inside book design by Dawn Von Strolley Grove

To John R. Lee, M.D., my friend, my mentor,
and a courageous medical pioneer,
and to my mother, Smiles Randolph,
who always believes in me,
my abilities, and my dreams with unconditional faith.

C.W.R.

CONTENTS

Acknowledgments...ix

Introduction: The Link Between Estrogen and Belly Fat xv

Part 1. Where Your Belly Fat Came From
    and Why It *Won't* Budge...1

  1. Estrogen Dominance:
    The Hidden Weight-Gain Epidemic 3
    Estrogen and Progesterone: A Careful
        Balancing Act...5
    What Is Estrogen Dominance?.................................6
    A Weight-Gain Double Whammy—How
        Your Body Becomes a "Fat Magnet" 7

  2. Are You Estrogen Dominant?.................................11
    Estrogen Dominance Self-Assessment.........................12
    Why the Symptoms Are Often Misdiagnosed.............19
    The Long-Term Health Risks of
        Estrogen Dominance 21

Part 2. The Three-Step Plan to Balance Your *Hormones* and Whittle Your Middle 23

3. Step 1: Eat Foods That Balance Your Hormones ..25

The Non-Negotiable Food List:

Foods That Reduce Estrogen Dominance 25

Other Foods to Add to Your Diet Every Day 30

Danger Zone: Foods and Drinks That

Increase Estrogen Levels 38

A Month of Hormone-Balancing Meal Plans 41

4. Step 2: Use Progesterone—the Simple Way to a Flat Belly 73

How to Safely and Effectively Boost

Declining Progesterone Levels 73

What Every Woman Needs to Know:

The Danger of Synthetic Hormones 74

Marketing a Dangerous Lie 77

How Bio-identical Progesterone Kick-Starts

Weight Loss at a Cellular Level 78

The Health Benefits of Bio-identical Progesterone 78

Forms of Bio-identical Progesterone 83

How to Use Progesterone on the Plan 84

What to Look for in a Progesterone Cream 85

5. Step 3: Take the Right Supplements to Support, Not Sabotage, Your Hormone Balance 89

Calcium D-Glucarate 89

Diindolylmethane (DIM) 90

The B Vitamins 90

Vitamin E..91

Calcium-Magnesium Combo 92

7-Keto Dehydroepiandrosterone (DHEA)............93

Chitosan...95

Part 3. Keeping That *Flat* Belly for Life 97

6. Keeping Weight Off in the Real World 99

Stress and Your Hormones 101

Sleep Disturbances and Your Hormones................110

Physical Inactivity and Your Hormones 111

Boosting Your Adrenal Glands.....................112

7. The 80-20 Rule...115

One Size Does Not Fit All 116

When You Will Need a Doctor 117

Why You Will Need a Compounding Pharmacy 118

8. The "Flat Belly for Life" Recipe Collection...........121

Main Dishes 122

Vegetable Dishes..151

Salads, Salad Dressings, and Snacks................171

Appendix A: Journal and Food Diary 191

Appendix B: How to Reduce the Estrogens in Your
     Environment..197

Appendix C: Resources.....................................201

References 218

Index 226

ACKNOWLEDGMENTS

This book would not have become a reality without the input, talent, and support of many individuals, including my coauthor, Genie James. Before I acknowledge each of them, however, I want to thank God for giving me the inspiration and courage to become both a physician and a healer. I am humbly aware that it is my privilege to serve as an instrument of our Creator. I also want to thank my mother, Smiles Randolph, for always believing in me and encouraging me to speak the truth.

I would not currently be regarded as a medical expert and a pioneer in the realm of bio-identical hormone replacement had it not been for my friend and mentor, the late John R. Lee, M.D., primary author of *What Your Doctor May Not Tell You About Perimenopause*, *What Your Doctor May Not Tell You About Menopause*, and *What Your Doctor May Not Tell You About Breast Cancer*. Dr. Lee's fingerprints remain on my heart and in my work.

In the medical and scientific fields, I would like to thank Joel Hargrove, M.D., for his willingness to oppose the pharmaceutical industry through his tenacity for groundbreaking medical research in the field of bio-identical hormone replacement; Christiane Northrup, M.D., for her unmistakable voice and published works that first helped to introduce the term *bio-identical* into the layperson's vocabulary; Erika Schwartz, M.D., for her strength and courage as a spokeswoman for our cause; Helene Leonetti, M.D., for research substantiating the clinical benefits of bio-identical progesterone replacement; Joann E. Manson, M.D., for her work in preventive medicine and hormone replacement; Kenna Stephenson, M.D., for her research examining how bio-identical hormone replacement positively influences women's cardiovascular health and aging process; James L. Wilson, N.D., for his illuminating work on the adrenal hormones; and David Zava, Ph.D., for his daring research linking breast cancer and synthetic hormone replacement.

I also want to acknowledge Virginia Hopkins for her pivotal role in working with Dr. Lee to coauthor the above-mentioned three books, which set the stage for the current revolution supporting the use of bio-identical hormone therapies. Since Dr. Lee's death, Ms. Hopkins continues her mission to educate the public about the safety and efficacy of bio-identical hormones through her website and newsletter.

Special kudos go to Colleen Reilly, executive director of Women in Balance, for her efforts to provide education on available research and for her willingness to address the confusion that healthcare providers express about hormone therapies—especially since the National Institutes of Health halted the Women's Health Initiative (WHI) study of synthetic hormone replacement therapy in postmenopausal women in July 2002.

Similarly, I applaud the leadership teams at the Professional Compounding Center of America (PCCA) and the International Association of Compounding Pharmacies (IACP) for their stamina in fighting the money-for-power exchange between pharmaceutical lobbyists and members of Congress. I am excited by the strides that these two organizations, along with Jim Paoletti (now at ZRT Laboratories), are making in educating the medical community on the safety and efficacy of bio-identical hormone replacement.

I have true gratitude for Nanette Noffsinger, our media and public relations consultant. Ms. Noffsinger represents us with a passion and an integrity that is inspiring. The fact that she could actually convince me to put on face powder before going before a camera is a testament to her gamut of skills!

Thanks are due to Susan Shee, our marketing coordinator and patient liaison for the Natural Hormone Institute of America. For more than a year, she patiently accomplished the day-to-day work, thereby allowing Ms. James to focus on this project. Others I would like to thank include John Kaszuba for his cutting-edge marketing talents and his help with our website and newsletter, as well as Mikel Taft and Jessica Vance, for their help typing, formatting, and walking the dogs when necessary. I also want to acknowledge Patti Landry, N.P., Anna Stauch, N.P., and Nicole Avens, N.P., Patti gracefully and firmly models the best of mind-body-spirit medicine; Anna blends extreme intelligence with sharp intuition as she cares for patients. Although Nicole is no longer with the practice, I continue to have the greatest admiration for her skills as an integrative medicine provider, particularly in the area of bio-identical hormone replacement. My entire office staff is incredible. It is because of their skills and commitment that we are able to serve a wide range of patients.

Finally, my deepest gratitude goes to my patients. Their weight-loss success stories created the framework for this book.

It has been a privilege to write this book. As a physician and a healer, I have always been grateful to serve one person at a time, but hours and logistics limit how many people one can touch or help in such a role. Thankfully, this book fulfills the mission to meet a wider breadth of need.

Even if you and I never meet or have a one-to-one conversation, perhaps you will embrace our three-step plan and, in doing so, save yourself a lifetime struggle with abdominal weight gain, other symptoms of hormone imbalance, and the risk of developing hormone-dependent cancers. Nothing brings me more joy than seeing patients living healthy, happy lives. I wish the same for you.

C.W. Randolph, Jr., M.D.

I am indebted to Pat Holdsworth, who evidenced a personal graciousness and tenacity that would ultimately characterize our entire publishing team at Health Communications. Most especially, I express deep thanks to Allison Janse and Michele Matrisciani for believing in the merit of this project and sharing their editing wisdom and enthusiasm for disseminating the truth.

Sincere appreciation also goes to Michelle Howry, now senior editor at Touchstone Fireside, because her input shifted the tone of this book and made it more accessible to the reader. I also thank Laura Yorke of the Carol Mann Agency for her initial contributions, her footwork, and her willingness to introduce us to a new realm of publishing.

Genie James

INTRODUCTION: THE LINK BETWEEN ESTROGEN AND BELLY FAT

I f you're a woman over thirty or a man over forty who has gained unwanted weight around your waist and belly, this book is for you. I hope to share information that will eliminate your guilt and feelings of resignation about your weight, and will also provide you with a solution. My premise, which is medically proven, is this: Those extra pounds that have crept up and become cemented around your middle have little to do with your inability to diet properly, limit carbs, or do crunches; they have everything to do with a shift in hormone production. In fact, belly fat is commonly the outward sign of a specific type of underlying hormone imbalance known as estrogen dominance.

As long as estrogen dominance remains unrecognized and untreated, your belly fat will be nearly impossible to lose, no

A Note to Readers: While this book was a team effort, it is written from Dr. Randolph's perspective, since he has treated thousands of patients. Through his hands-on experience as a physician, he uncovered the link between estrogen and belly fat.

matter what you do or how hard you try. Fortunately, estrogen dominance can be eliminated almost effortlessly, and once hormone balance is restored, the pounds that are attached to your middle will start to melt away without food deprivation or calorie counting.

How do I know this? As a physician, I have focused my life's work on how to safely and effectively reestablish optimal hormonal balance, mostly in women. I graduated from Auburn University's School of Pharmacy in 1971 and worked as a licensed compounding pharmacist before returning to school to become a physician. I received my medical degree from Louisiana State University School of Medicine in 1982 and my board certification in obstetrics and gynecology in 1986.

Over the past decade, my professional expertise has expanded to include a focus on natural, or integrative, medicine. In 2000, I attended a continuing medical education program at Columbia University Medical School, where I completed intensive training under Andrew Weil, M.D. In 2005, I became a board-certified Diplomate of the American Board of Holistic Medicine. It humbles me that after more than two decades of clinical practice, I am internationally recognized as a pioneer in the field of bio-identical hormone replacement therapies (BHRT). *Bio-identical* refers to plant-derived hormone molecules that are identical to the natural human hormones produced by the body.

the cure for the "bloated belly" syndrome

For years, women have sought my help as a physician because they knew something wasn't right. They came to my office suffering from symptoms such as hot flashes, night sweats, irregular bleeding, bloating, memory loss, low libido, and mood swings. In almost every case, these women also evidenced another unwanted side effect: abdominal weight gain. They used all sorts of terms to describe their extra weight: "pooching tummy," "bloated belly," "pregnant stomach," or even "that new continent that has attached itself to my hips." Men who realized that something was shifting with their hormones also sought help. Most often, male patients' primary symptoms would be loss of sex drive, fatigue, and depression. The fact that these men almost always had a spare tire was just part of the presenting package.

During the patients' physical examinations, I would most always write "increased abdominal circumference" on their medical charts. Then, without paying any more attention to their weight, I would move on to address what I considered a more pressing concern: how their health was being sabotaged by shifting hormone production and, subsequently, an underlying condition of estrogen dominance. I wasn't aware then of the link between hormone levels and the size of a person's waist.

Based on my background in pharmacology and medical training, I developed a holistic approach to treat this condition of estrogen dominance. The approach has three components:

1. A diet specifically designed to reduce the body's estrogen levels.
2. Natural hormone replacement therapy to restore hormone equilibrium.
3. A select list of vitamins and supplements that have been proven to work synergistically to support optimal hormone balance.

the results

After following the plan, hormone balance was restored in all of my patients, and their symptoms of estrogen dominance disappeared. Their overall health improved usually within one or two months. But, surprisingly, within a week or two, most patients enjoyed an additional benefit: those stubborn pounds they carried around for years began to melt away, and their bellies went from bloated to flat! Within several months, many patients came to me, requesting what they called the "belly-flat diet."

I soon realized that this plan could help many people beyond the scope of my medical practice. So, I elicited the help of Genie James, the coauthor of my first book, *From Hormone Hell to Hormone Well,* the cofounder of the Natural Hormone Institute of America, also my wife. Not only does she have a Masters of Medical Science from Emory University, she has a distinct expertise in the fields of women's health and complementary medicine.

Once we shared the plan publicly, we saw tremendous results. In general, men and women who committed to the diet saw exciting results in just three to four weeks. A typical first-month response was a loss of four to seven pounds. More important, most waistlines shrank by one to two inches in the first few weeks.

By the second month, the pounds and inches dropped even faster, because once hormonal equilibrium was reestablished, the body's metabolism picked up and burned even more calories for energy.

And although the primary goal of this book is to eliminate the underlying condition of estrogen dominance that is causing unwanted weight gain, the benefits of the plan extend beyond the cosmetic; innumerable medical studies also link estrogen dominance with several potentially lethal health risks.

If you stay on the plan indefinitely, it will have a long-term positive impact on your overall health and well being. It will give you a lifetime of balanced hormones, a flat belly, and better health. Is there any reason you should not get started today?

1

WHERE YOUR BELLY FAT CAME FROM AND WHY IT *won't* BUDGE

My guess is that you picked up this book because, over the last few years, you have put on ten, twenty, thirty, or even forty extra pounds around your abdomen, hips, and thighs. The extra weight makes you feel uncomfortable and unattractive. You've tried dieting and exercising to lose the belly fat, and while you may have lost a few pounds here and there for short periods of time, the bulk of your extra weight just hangs on.

In Part 1, you'll learn the medical reason why your belly fat appeared and why it just won't budge, no matter how hard you try. In Chapter 1, you'll learn how hormone balance is intricately connected with your body's metabolism and its predisposition to store fat. Even more important, you'll come to understand why estrogen dominance is very likely the primary hidden culprit adding pounds to your belly and inches to your waist. Already wondering if you might be estrogen dominant? In Chapter 2, you'll learn how to self-diagnose the problem.

ESTROGEN DOMINANCE: THE HIDDEN WEIGHT-GAIN EPIDEMIC

When people hear the term *hormonal imbalance*, most immediately think about the change of life, menopause. Although it's true that women going through menopause have significant hormonal changes, the issues associated with hormonal imbalance, such as abdominal weight gain, typically begin in a woman's early to mid-thirties and a man's early forties.

In fact, weight-loss research proves that because of shifting hormone production, the average person will add one to two pounds around his or her middle each year between the ages of thirty-five and fifty-five. As long as your body's cellular metabolism is compromised by an untreated hormone imbalance—most particularly estrogen dominance—the extra pounds around your middle will be nearly impossible to lose.

I firmly believe that estrogen dominance is an epidemic in North America. We Americans are aging, we are constantly exposed to environmental estrogens, and too many of us are overweight.

Unfortunately, because the pharmaceutical industry has created so much marketing hype about a woman's need for estrogen replacement as a fountain-of-youth treatment for menopause, most medical practitioners and healthcare consumers are misinformed and/or confused. The consequence for millions of people is that the very real condition of estrogen dominance is often overlooked or, worse, misdiagnosed and mistreated. For instance, consider the case of a woman I'll call Sylvia.

Sylvia, a thirty-six-year-old divorced mother of three, came to my office six months after moving to Florida from Oregon. She said that she had gained twenty-five pounds in three years and was suffering from what she called the "love-handle blues." She was in tears as she explained the following:

> *Ever since my divorce three years ago, I have felt as if someone was pumping up a spare tire around my middle. I used to wear size 6 pants, and now I can barely squeeze into size 10. I swear I'm not eating any more than I did five years ago. If anything, I eat less. Even though I go to the gym and walk on a treadmill at least five hours a week, this fat around my belly just won't budge.*
>
> *I can't go on this way. I am almost at the point of considering diet pills. Also, my doctor on the West Coast had put me on antidepressants, but my prescription has expired. Please help me.*

Sylvia's age, weight gain, and mild depression were common indicators of an underlying hormonal imbalance, specifically estrogen dominance. I told Sylvia that I could help her without diet pills or antidepressants. After following the plan for six weeks, she walked into the office a changed woman. She had lost nine pounds and an inch and a half from her waist. Within ten weeks, she celebrated with a shopping spree for new size 8 pants. In my practice, I have helped thousands of people like Sylvia, people who had no idea that shifting hormone production was the hidden culprit causing their weight gain.

In order for you to understand how a hormone imbalance could affect your weight, here's a quick refresher course in the production and function of your sex hormones.

estrogen and progesterone: a careful balancing act

The human body produces three sex hormones: estrogen, progesterone, and testosterone. In this book I focus primarily on estrogen and progesterone because both medical research and my experience prove that they play the starring roles in any hormone-related weight-gain drama.

healthy hormone function from puberty to thirty

When a woman begins to menstruate until she is approximately thirty years old, her ratio of estrogen to progesterone is optimal. In this ideal scenario, estrogen does the following for her:

- Develops the sex organs and secondary sex characteristics such as breasts and pubic hair.
- Maintains the menstrual cycle.
- Supports the growth and function of the uterus, specifically creating the lining of the uterus to prepare it for pregnancy.
- Stimulates cell growth.

During these same years, progesterone does the following:

- Maintains the uterus and prepares it for pregnancy during the reproductive years.
- Promotes the survival of an ovum (egg) once it is fertilized.
- Stimulates bone building that can prevent or treat osteoporosis.
- Acts as a natural diuretic to prevent bloating.

In women and men, progesterone also does the following:

- Serves as a natural antidepressant.
- Fosters a calming effect on the body.
- Maintains libido.
- Promotes regular sleep patterns.
- Opposes estrogen's predisposition to promote cell growth, thereby providing protection from uterine, breast, and ovarian cancer as well as fibrocystic disease in females and an increased risk of prostate cancer in males.

As you can see, when they are in sync, estrogen and progesterone are responsible for important biochemical functions in both the female and male bodies. When the ratio of estrogen and progesterone gets out of sync, many health issues arise, including unwanted weight gain.

what is estrogen dominance?

It is important to understand that being estrogen dominant doesn't mean that your body is producing too much estrogen;

rather, it means that your body's estrogen production is not balanced by progesterone production. Estrogen dominance occurs when the natural ratio of estrogen to progesterone is upset—in other words, when the body's internal estrogen-to-progesterone seesaw becomes tilted.

a weight-gain double whammy—how your body becomes a "fat magnet"

Estrogen dominance causes a host of metabolic distur bances, which occur much like a chicken-and-egg relationship:

- Too much estrogen circulating in the body increases body fat, and fatty tissue within the body produces and stores more estrogen. Body fat contains an enzyme that converts adrenal steroids to estrogen. At a cellular level, body fat continues to produce more estrogen, and a high estrogen level, in turn, causes the body to increase its store of fatty tissue. In other words, your belly becomes a "fat magnet."

- When you're estrogen dominant, your body is unable to effectively use fat stores for energy, which means that your body's ability to metabolize or burn body fat for calories is compromised. The result is extra weight that won't go away even with more exercise or less eating.

- When high estrogen levels are unopposed by sufficient progesterone, the resulting condition of estrogen dom-inance also impacts your body fat's distribution. In both men and women, higher estrogen levels predispose the body to store fat around the abdomen. In women, estrogen dominance causes fat to be stored around the waist, hips, and thighs, and it's the main reason that many middle-age women have pear-shaped bodies. Estrogen dominance is also the reason for the middle-age spare tire in men.

Hormonal Imbalance

Estrogen Dominance

Increased Estrogen Dominance

Weight Gain/Belly Fat Produces More Estrogen

effects on the thyroid gland

The thyroid gland is best known for its metabolic function affecting weight. Estrogen dominance renders the thyroid hormones dysfunctional, causing your body's metabolism to slow down. The resulting condition is called *relative hypothyroidism*. In addition, the changes in your body's blood sugar levels—some of which occur naturally with age and some of which are due to a hormone imbalance—are also linked to weight gain. As the body's progesterone production decreases with age and estrogen becomes dominant, your body releases insulin more rapidly and more often. When fluctuating hormones unnaturally stimulate insulin release, you get hungry faster and will often crave sugar. In fact, these food cravings can sometimes be uncontrollable, and people who are estrogen dominant tend to consume more sweets even when they aren't truly hungry. As a result, they ingest more calories than their bodies require and pack on even more pounds.

If you are a woman in your thirties, you need to understand that estrogen dominance is not "your mother's problem." For most women, estrogen dominance is a concern to be reckoned with long before middle age or menopause. As a woman approaches her midthirties, the balance of hormones within her body begins to shift, starting with a decline in progesterone. In fact, progesterone production declines 120 times more rapidly than does estrogen production. It is this downward shift in progesterone production that causes the body to become estrogen dominant.

Contrary to the popular belief that estrogen is solely a female hormone, men can also be estrogen dominant. In men, progesterone is produced in the adrenal and testicular tissue. When men reach their forties, falling progesterone levels lead to a fall in testosterone levels. As both the progesterone and testosterone levels decline, the male body becomes estrogen dominant. To find out if estrogen dominance is responsible for your increased belly fat—and possibly a host of other physical, mental, and emotional concerns and health risks—continue reading. Chapter 2 will help you to understand how age, body fat, and environmental toxins can join forces to sabotage your inner hormonal equilibrium.

ARE YOU ESTROGEN DOMINANT?

Evelyn, a thirty-seven-year-old graphic artist and mother of three, walked into my office literally dragging her forty-three-year-old husband, Richard, behind her. I had delivered all three of her children and had been her gynecologist for years. Evelyn related the following:

> Dr. Randolph, remember how trim and athletic my body was even after three kids? Even two years ago, I was a perfect size 8. Now I am a size 12 and I look like I swallowed a bowling ball.
>
> I am still relatively young. I'm not even forty, but I feel like I am living in a stranger's body. And I am not the only one. Until three years ago, he [pointing to Richard] could wear the same golfing pants he wore in college. Now he's gained thirty pounds in the last four years.
>
> I cook all the same foods I have for the past fifteen years, so I know it's not a change in our diet. I still go to an aerobics class every other morning and play tennis three times a week. So what could it be? Just old age?

Evelyn and Richard were both experiencing estrogen dominance and were exhibiting "flashing red light" symptoms and behaviors. To determine if you might be estrogen dominant, answer the four questions below.

ESTROGEN DOMINANCE SELF-ASSESSMENT

❏ Question 1: How Old Are You?

If you are a woman older than thirty or a man older than forty, (men, see page 13 for further details) you are most likely estrogen dominant.

As mentioned in the last chapter, a woman's progesterone level begins to decline in her thirties, even while the ovaries are still producing enough estrogen to stimulate the monthly cycle. From early or midthirties through mid- or late forties, a woman who is regularly menstruating is said to be premenopausal. When a woman's periods become irregular—in some cases skipping months at a time and in other cases becoming heavy and flooding—she is said to be perimenopausal. In this stage of life, the ovaries' production of estrogen is also declining, but progesterone production continues to decline even more significantly. The result is continual estrogen dominance.

Even during and after menopause, estrogen dominance is still a concern. The average age of a woman entering natural menopause in the United States is fifty-one years old. Many women make the mistake of thinking that if they are no longer menstruating, they no longer have to worry about the levels of hormones that are circulating in their bodies. This is wrong. It is a misconception to believe that when a woman stops having periods, her ovaries turn off like a light switch.

Although menopause indicates a drastic shift in your body's hormonal equilibrium, it does not mean that the sex hormones are suddenly absent from your body. The ovaries of a menopausal woman are still quite actively producing 40 to 60 percent of the estrogen produced by a premenopausal woman. Progesterone production, however, continues to decline. The result is that many menopausal and postmenopausal women continue to suffer from estrogen dominance.

Approximately one in every four American women will enter an abrupt, artificial menopause as the result of a hysterectomy. If you are a woman who has had a partial hysterectomy—that is, removal of the uterus only—you can still be estrogen dominant because your ovaries will continue to produce some estrogen and even less progesterone.

If you are a woman who has had a complete hysterectomy—that is, removal of the entire reproductive tract (the uterus, fallopian tubes, and ovaries), you can still be estrogen dominant. Even though you no longer have ovaries, your body fat is still producing estrogen.

Estrogen-Dominant Men

For men, *Question 1* is easy. If you are a man older than forty, your progesterone and testosterone levels have already started to decline. If you feel sluggish, bloated, and/or lethargic, these are symptoms of an underlying hormonal imbalance. Your age and your symptoms indicate that you are in the midst of male menopause, or andropause. Decreased sexual appetite, abdominal weight gain, and an inability to lose weight are three indications that you are most likely estrogen dominant.

❏ Question 2: How Long Have You Been Overweight?

If you have been ten pounds overweight for a year or more, you are most likely caught in the cycle of increasing estrogen dominance. As described in Chapter 1, high estrogen levels cause you to develop more fatty tissue in your body, which in turn produces more estrogen in your body.

❏ Question 3: Do You Have Symptoms of Estrogen Dominance?

Weight gain is only one symptom of an underlying hormone imbalance. Because hormone receptors are located throughout the body and in the brain, estrogen dominance can manifest in a host of physical, emotional, and mental ailments. These include anxiety, depression, fatigue, breast tenderness, headaches (including migraines), digestive disorders, fuzzy thinking and/or memory loss, and low libido. Look at the box on page 15. If two or more of these symptoms apply to you, and if these symptoms have been present for more than three months, it is likely a signal that you are suffering from an underlying condition of estrogen dominance.

Symptoms of Hormone Imbalance

Women	Men
Mood swings	Burned out feeling
Hot flashes	Abdominal fat
Night sweats	Prostate problems
Fatigue	Decreased mental clarity
Headaches	Decreased sex drive
Depressed	Increased urinary urge
Anxious	Decreased strength
Nervous	Decreased stamina
Irritable	Difficulty sleeping
Tearful	Decreased urine flow
Memory lapse	Irritable
Weight gain	Depressed
Premature aging	Erectile dysfunction
Vaginal dryness	Night sweats
Heavy menses	Poor concentration
Bleeding changes	
Incontinence	
Fibrocystic breasts	
Decreased sex drive	
Tender breasts	
Osteoporosis	
Water retention	

❑ Question 4: Does Your Environment Put You at Risk?

Simply living in an industrialized nation puts you at risk for estrogen dominance. However, if you are in a work situation where you are constantly being exposed to toxic fumes or if your home is located near a toxic waste dump, the chances that your environment is contributing to your condition of estrogen dominance is even greater.

Environmental estrogen, or xenoestrogen (pronounced "ZEE-no-estrogen"), can be found in pesticides, herbicides, fungicides, plastics, fuels, car exhausts, dry cleaning chemicals, industrial waste, and meat from animals that have been fed estrogenic drugs to fatten them. It is also found in the synthetic estrogen and progesterone (chemically termed *progestin*) of birth control pills and hormone therapies; these synthetic hormones are secreted in women's urine, are flushed down the toilet, and eventually make their way back into the food chain. Over time, these foreign estrogens can dangerously accumulate and increase the estrogen load in the body.

People living in the United States and in western Europe have been found to have much higher estrogen levels at much younger ages than people living in less industrialized countries. Many experts link these high levels of estrogen to environmental exposure. Estrogen-like hormones in the foods we eat and the chemicals we use every day are often hidden causes of estrogen dominance. These estrogen-like hormones mimic the action of the estrogen produced in our bodies. We are exposed to them through certain chemicals (xenoestrogens) and through specific types of foods and plants (phytoestrogens).

Although most of our exposure to xenoestrogens comes in small amounts, the problem is that most of us are exposed to many tiny doses every day, which has a dangerous, cumulative effect.

Chronic exposure to environmental estrogens can contribute to estrogen dominance occurring at a much younger age. The increasing number of younger women who are experiencing anovulatory menstrual cycles is a silent signal of estrogen dominance. An anovulatory cycle is a cycle in which ovulation fails to occur, which means that a woman bleeds but doesn't release an egg, or ovulate. Anovulatory cycles occur when a woman's body isn't making enough progesterone to balance the estrogen that builds up the uterine lining. Medical studies have shown that by age thirty-five, approximately 50 percent of women are having anovulatory cycles.

Even women and men in their teens and twenties have been found to suffer from estrogen dominance that stems from environmental exposure. The symptoms include weight gain, PMS, fibrocystic breasts, bloating, troublesome periods, infertility, endometriosis, depression, and mood swings.

Xenoestrogens

Xeno literally means foreign; therefore, xenoestrogens are foreign estrogens. In addition to being highly estrogenic, xenoestrogens are fat soluble and nonbiodegradable. This means that they easily pass through the skin and sit in fatty tissues and that they don't break down over time, in either the body or the environment. Some common sources of xenoestrogens include:

Meat and dairy products. In the United States, most ranchers inject their cattle and sheep with synthetic steroid growth-promoting hormones. Hormone-treated meat is a very real health issue. In the late nineties, Roy Hertz, then director of endocrinology at the National Cancer Institute and a leading authority on hormonal cancers, warned of the carcinogenic risks of estrogenic additives, which can cause imbalances in natural hormone levels.

Pesticides and plastics. Chemical pesticides, herbicides, and fungicides are routinely applied to mass-produced fruits and vegetables. In addition, most people routinely use bug sprays, weed killers, and other pesticides in their homes and yards. Finally, plastic products are part of almost every person's daily life, and many of them give off xenoestrogens when heated, whether purposely in a microwave oven or accidentally in a hot car.

Petrochemicals and solvents. Many general hygiene products—such as skin cream, lotion, soap, shampoo, perfume, hair spray, and room deodorizers—contain petrochemicals. These compounds often have chemical structures similar to estrogen and therefore act like estrogen when introduced into the body. Industrial solvents are another source of xenoestrogens and are commonly found in cosmetics, fingernail polish, fingernail polish remover, glue, paint, varnish, cleaning products, carpet, fiberboard, and other processed woods.

Synthetic hormone replacement drugs and birth control pills. Synthetic hormone repla cement drugs such as Premarin, Prempro, Femhrt, Menest, Ortho-Est, Activella, and many other brand names, as well as birth control pills, contribute to the development or worsening of estrogen dominance.

Many doctors routinely continue to prescribe synthetic hormone replacement therapy for menopausal symptoms, such as hot flashes, night sweats, insomnia, and moodiness. These prescription drugs are composed of synthetic estrogen or a synthetic estrogen and progestin combination. Synthetic hormone replacement has also been prescribed to protect women from the loss of bone mass after menopause.

More than a decade ago, we became convinced that natural bio-identical hormone replacement therapy (BHRT) was a safer and more effective option for treating the symptoms of hormone imbalance than synthetic hormones manufactured and marketed by large pharmaceutical companies. In fact, our first book, *From Hormone Hell to Hormone Well*, focused on the benefits of BHRT versus synthetic hormone therapies.

Like synthetic hormone replacement pills, birth control pills also contain synthetic estrogen and progestin. Depending on dosage, they can be very potent and linger in the body for a long time. Birth control pills work by keeping estrogen at such a falsely high level that the body is fooled into responding as if it were pregnant. Therefore, ovulation does not occur. Chapter 3 addresses the dangers of synthetic hormones in greater detail.

why the symptoms are often misdiagnosed

When Sylvia in Chapter 1 first complained of the "love-handle blues," her previous doctor responded by giving her a prescription for antidepressants. Unfortunately, the inappropriate use of antidepressants to treat estrogen dominance is far too common. In recent years, more than 70 percent of the prescriptions written for the type of antidepressant called selective serotonin reuptake inhibitors (SSRIs) came from primary care and ob-gyn physicians—that is, physicians who have no special training in mental health disorders!

Genie was working as a pharmaceutical representative for Eli Lilly in 1987 when the company launched the first SSRI, Prozac. During sales meetings, she was instructed to target ob-gyns and sell them on Prozac as a cure for the symptoms of premenstrual syndrome (PMS), such as depression, mood swings, bloating, and anxiety. Evidently, the recommended sales technique worked. Prozac soon accounted for one-quarter of Lilly's revenues, with annual sales reaching $2.6 billion.

In 2000, just before Prozac was to lose its patent protection in 2001, Eli Lilly changed the name from Prozac to Sarafem, changed the pill's color from green and white to pink and lavender, and got FDA approval to market it for severe premenstrual symptoms, or premenstrual dysphoric disorder (PMDD). Prior to the launch of Sarafem, Lilly spent $2.3 billion on marketing, much more than the $1.5 billion it had spent on the drug's research and development.

It saddens me to realize that many women (and men) who tell their physicians that they suffer from moodiness and mild depression leave their doctor's office with a prescription for an antidepressant while their underlying condition of estrogen dominance remains unrecognized and untreated. Unlike antidepressant drugs or manufactured synthetic hormones, bio-identical hormone therapies cannot be patented. Therefore, there are no company sales representatives going into physicians' offices to educate them about the causes and dangers of estrogen dominance.

Because of this ignorance within the medical community, many women and men continue to suffer needlessly. Worst of all, when a woman complains of even the slightest symptoms of estrogen dominance, most conventional medical doctors recommend a prescription of synthetic estrogen replacement. This practice is both irresponsible and dangerous, and even though it is usually rooted in ignorance, it can have tragic consequences.

the long-term health risks of estrogen dominance

The relationship between estrogen dominance and weight gain is a very real concern, but there are others as well. Clinical studies conducted in both the United States and Europe link estrogen dominance to many other health risks. For instance, in both men and women, estrogen-related belly fat is a contributing risk factor for developing cardiovascular disease. According to the Food and Drug Administration (FDA), women with a waist measurement of more than thirty-five inches and men with a waist measurement of more than forty inches are very likely to be at risk.

Estrogen also fuels cell growth, and unchecked cell growth, or proliferation, is a precursor for cancer. In women, elevated estrogen levels have been linked to an increased risk for endometriosis and fibroids as well as breast and uterine hormone-dependent cancers. (In hormone-dependent cancers, a tumor requires hormones, specifically estrogen, in order to grow. The medical term for such tumors is *estrogen receptor-positive*.) In men, estrogen dominance has been linked to an increased risk of hormone-dependent prostate cancer.

An increasing number of studies link exposure to environmental estrogens to an increased risk of cancer. In her book *The Truth About Breast Cancer*, Claire Hoy states the following:

> *Greenpeace found that one country that banned pesticides—Israel—quickly went from breast cancer rates that were among the highest in the world to rates in keeping with other industrialized nations. It also found that U.S. counties with chemical waste sites were 6.5 times more likely to have elevated breast cancer rates than those without waste sites.*

After reading this chapter, you should be able to determine if your age, your body fat, your symptoms, and your chronic exposure to environmental estrogens signal that you are suffering from estrogen dominance. If your situation and symptoms fit, then stop feeling guilty about those extra pounds around your middle. They are not your fault. At a cellular level, you have been, and continue to be, set up.

Nevertheless, don't give up. You can eliminate your condition of estrogen dominance once and for all while having a very positive impact on your overall health and well-being. The next few chapters will tell you exactly how.

PART 2

THE THREE-STEP PLAN TO BALANCE YOUR *hormones* AND WHITTLE YOUR MIDDLE

The next three chapters will provide you with the details of the three-step plan to balance your hormones and help you acquire the flat belly that goes with it. Chapter 3 describes the foods that will help to decrease your body's estrogen load. Chapter 4 explains how to safely and effectively boost your body's declining progesterone levels without a prescription. Chapter 5 provides a list of supplements you can take to support overall hormone balance.

STEP 1:
EAT FOODS THAT BALANCE YOUR HORMONES

A complaint I hear many times a day is "I try to eat a low-calorie, low-fat diet and I exercise regularly, but no matter what I do, those pounds around my middle just won't budge." Does this sound familiar?

With an awareness of how certain foods can help to decrease the body's estrogen load, we have developed a diet, moderately high in calories, that allows for protein and healthy fats at every meal. It includes ample portions of "belly-blaster" foods that will reduce or eliminate your extra estrogen load.

THE NON-NEGOTIABLE FOOD LIST: FOODS THAT REDUCE ESTROGEN DOMINANCE

The stars of the nutritional component of the plan are cruciferous vegetables, citrus fruits, insoluble fiber, and lignans, because these foods function within your body to reduce an unhealthy estrogen load.

Belly Blaster 1: Cruciferous Vegetables
Benefit to your body: indole-3-carbinol (I3C)
✓ EAT 2–3 SERVINGS PER DAY.

Cruciferous vegetables are a critical part of your success on this plan. Eating large amounts of broccoli, asparagus, cauliflower, spinach, Brussels sprouts, celery, beet root, kale, cabbage, parsley root, radish, turnip, collard greens, and mustard greens have been shown to improve the production of "good" estrogen. Although not considered cruciferous, asparagus and spinach are also "belly blasters" because they also improve "good" estrogen levels.

There are three kinds of natural estrogens: estrone (E1), estradiol (E2), and estriol (E3). All estrogens tend to promote cell division, but unchecked cell division can lead to cancer. E2 is the most stimulating to breast and uterine tissues, and E1 is less so; thus, they might be called the "bad" estrogens. In contrast, E3 may be thought of as the "good" estrogen because medical studies have shown that it protects us from cancer. Cruciferous vegetables contain a phytonutrient called indole-3-carbinol (I3C), which has been shown to act as a catalyst to decrease the body's load of "bad" estrogens. These vegetables therefore help to reduce estrogen dominance.

If you're not a fan of cruciferous vegetables, try some of the recipes in Chapter 8. You just might become a cauliflower convert!

Belly Blaster 2: Citrus Fruits
Benefit to your body: d-Limonene
✓ EAT 1 SERVING PER DAY.

A substance called d-Limonene, which is found in the oils of citrus fruits, has been shown to promote the detoxification of estrogen. Common citrus fruits are oranges, grapefruit, tangerines, lemons, limes, and tangelos. Research has also found that when male and female lab mice were administered an extract of d-Limonene, they lost weight.

Belly Blaster 3: Insoluble Fiber
Benefit to your body: estrogen binder
✓ EAT 2 SERVINGS PER DAY.

There are two types of fiber: soluble and insoluble. Soluble fiber dissolves in water and is degraded by bacteria in your colon. It forms a gel in your intestines that regulates the flow of waste material through your digestive tract. This type of fiber is found in oatmeal, oat bran, dried peas, beans, lentils, apples, pears, strawberries, and blueberries. Soluble fiber is good for you, but no matter how much of it you eat, it won't influence your hormonal equilibrium. Insoluble fiber, on the other hand, can directly help to decrease estrogen overload. It binds itself to extra estrogen in the digestive tract, which is then excreted by the body. Sources of insoluble fiber are any whole grains—whole-wheat bread, barley, couscous, brown rice, whole-grain cereal, and wheat bran—as well as seeds, carrots, cucumbers, zucchini, celery, and tomatoes.

Belly Blaster 4: Lignans
Benefit to your body: estrogen binder
✓ EAT 2–3 TABLESPOONS PER DAY.

Ground or milled flaxseed, sesame seeds, and flaxseed oil are part of a food group called *lignans*. The friendly bacteria in our intestines convert plant lignans into a substance that has a weak estrogen-like activity. When there are low estrogen levels in your body, these weak lignan estrogens make up for some of the deficiency. When the body is estrogen dominant, however, these lignan estrogens bind to your body's estrogen receptors, thereby reducing human estrogen activity at a cellular level.

You can get your daily lignan benefit by adding the above mentioned foods to smoothies, yogurt, or salads. Sesame seed oil (tahini) also makes a delicious salad dressing when mixed with lemon juice, garlic, and water in a blender.

Table 3-1 gives a list of the four belly-blasting food groups and recommended daily amounts.

Table 3-1. Foods That Reduce Your Estrogen Load

Food Group	Servings/Day	Comments
CRUCIFEROUS VEGETABLES (½ CUP COOKED) ❖ Broccoli ❖ Arugula ❖ Cauliflower ❖ Brussels sprouts ❖ Celery ❖ Beet root ❖ Kale ❖ Cabbage ❖ Parsley root ❖ Radish ❖ Turnip, collard, or mustard greens ❖ Bok choy ❖ Rutabagas ❖ Asparagus ❖ Spinach	2–3	Cruciferous vegetables should be cooked by steaming, stir frying, baking, or boiling. Raw cruciferous vegetables contain thyroid inhibitors known as *goitrogens*. Eating excessive amounts of raw cruciferous vegetables has been linked to hypothyroid disease. If you want to eat cruciferous vegetables raw, limit to 2–3 servings per week.
CITRUS FRUITS ❖ 1 medium orange ❖ ½ grapefruit ❖ 2 tangerines ❖ 1–2 tangelos ❖ 2 Lemons ❖ 2 Limes	1	For a single serving, you may substitute ¾ cup of 100% fruit juice once every other day.

Table 3-1. Foods That Reduce Your Estrogen Load (cont'd)

Food Group	Servings/Day	Comments
INSOLUBLE FIBER ❖ ½ cup cooked whole grains or whole-wheat pasta ❖ 1 slice whole-wheat bread ❖ ½ cup cooked barley ❖ ½ cup cooked couscous ❖ ½ cup cooked brown rice ❖ ½ cup whole-grain cereal, such as kasha ❖ ½ cup wheat bran ❖ ½ cup pumpkin seeds ❖ ½ cup cooked carrots or 1 cup raw carrots ❖ 1 cup sliced cucumbers ❖ ½ cup cooked zucchini ❖ 1 cup raw celery ❖ 1 medium tomato	2	Read the labels. Some products with "whole-wheat" on the label will be made not with whole grains but with white flour and caramel coloring. Many people make the mistake of thinking that whole-grain products are fattening. They are not unless you add butter or creamy toppings. Leave these off. Healthier seasoning alternatives will be provided in the recipes.
LIGNANS ❖ Flaxseed or sesame seeds ❖ Flaxseed oil	2–3 tablespoons	Stir into low-fat yogurt or cottage cheese or sprinkle atop steamed vegetables.

OTHER FOODS TO ADD TO YOUR DIET EVERY DAY

A unique feature of this diet is that the food groups work in concert to support optimal hormonal equilibrium, provide energy, and promote good health as the pounds melt away. In addition to the belly-blasting foods, you should add the following foods to your daily diet.

Protein

✓ EAT 1 SERVING WITH EVERY MEAL.

Your body needs protein every day. Protein contains the essential amino acids that are required by the body for growth and for the maintenance of lean muscle tissue. In addition, according to a study published in the *Journal of Cell Metabolism*, a high-protein diet can also increase the amount of a hunger-fighting hormone circulating within the body. The hormone, known as peptide YY (or PYY), had already been found by the researchers to reduce food intake by a third when it was administered by injection to both normal-weight and obese people.

Rachel Batterham, the clinical scientist who led the study, said, "We've now found that increasing the protein content of the diet augments the body's own PYY, helping to reduce hunger and aid weight loss."

High-protein foods slow the movement of food from the stomach to the intestines. Slower stomach emptying means that you feel full longer and get hungrier later. In addition, protein has a gentle, steady effect on blood sugar, as opposed to the quick, steep rise in blood sugar caused by carbohydrates like white bread, cookies, or a baked potato. Finally, the body uses more energy (i.e., calories) to digest protein than it does to digest fat or carbohydrates.

Fish is a great source of protein. Salmon, trout, herring, water-packed tuna, and mackerel are also excellent sources of omega-3 fatty acids, which medical studies have found to have a strong cardiovascular benefit. Due to the health hazards associated with xenoestrogens that were mentioned in Chapter 2, we urge you to eat only organic meats and poultry, which are produced without chemicals or growth hormones.

Even with organic meats, some choices are better sources of protein than others. Red meat is usually higher in fat, particularly saturated fat. There are, however, plenty of lean complete proteins, including the breast meat of poultry and eggs from organic, free-running hens.

Organic plant sources of protein such as beans, legumes, and nuts are also excellent choices, but plant proteins must be combined in order to form a complete protein (e.g., rice and beans).

You should eat a serving of protein with every meal. Table 3-2 lists some good protein sources.

Table 3-2. Protein Sources and Serving Sizes

Protein Source	Serving Size	Comments
Fish	6 ounces	Steam, bake, grill, or stir-fry in olive oil. Do not fry.
Poultry	6 ounces	Skinless breast meat has the lowest fat.
Eggs	1 large	Boil, scramble, or poach.
Black beans	1 cup	Combine with rice for a complete protein.
Veggie burger	1 patty	(See recipe in Chapter 8.)
Chickpeas	1 cup	Buy canned and heat or soak dry chickpeas for 24 hours before cooking.
Dried beans: lima, black-eyed peas, lentils	1 cup	Buy canned and heat, or soak dry beans for 24 hours before cooking.
Tree nuts: almonds, pecans, walnuts, Brazil nuts	1/4 cup	Best raw or roasted. Avoid heavily salted or honey-roasted nuts.
Lean red meats	4 ounces	Limit to once per week.

Calcium

✓ EAT 2 SERVINGS EVERY DAY.

The body's need for calcium becomes increasingly pertinent for women and men as they age. Human bones replace about one-fifth of their total calcium each year, and there is a constant movement of calcium in and out of the bones, both for repair and to maintain a constant level of calcium in the blood and in other body fluids.

A big bonus for the premenopausal or perimenopausal woman is that calcium has been shown to reduce the abdominal cramping and the muscular contractions that result from PMS. Calcium is even more important for women who are approaching menopause or who are in the midst of it, because calcium helps to put the brakes on the development of osteoporosis, a debilitating bone disorder that causes brittle bones and a bent or stooped stance. Osteoporosis is a virtual epidemic among American women past the age of sixty, and it results from the body having insufficient calcium.

Men, too, need calcium. The body, regardless of gender, requires a certain amount of calcium to flow through its blood and soft tissues every day in order for the muscles to contract correctly, the blood to clot, and the nerves to carry messages. When men don't get adequate amounts of dietary calcium, their bodies meet their calcium needs by stealing the mineral from their bones. This weakens the bones over time and contributes to the development of osteoporosis. Although most people think of calcium deficiency as a woman's problem, of the 25 million Americans with osteoporosis, one in five is a man. The percentage rises as age increases, so that after the age of seventy-five, 50 percent of those affected are men.

Products made with milk are a great source of calcium; however, there might be hormones in your milk that can cause you harm. In 1994, the FDA approved the use of a bovine growth hormone called recombinant bovine somatotropin (rBST). According to rBST manufacturers, injections of this hormone cause a cow to produce up to 20 percent more milk. The growth hormone also stimulates the cow's liver to increase insulin-like growth factor 1 (IGF-1). Excess levels of IGF-1 have been increasingly linked by modern research to human cancer development and growth.

Recently, the pharmaceutical company Eli Lilly, a manufacturer of rBST, reported a tenfold increase in IGF-1 levels in the milk of cows that had been injected with the hormone. IGF-1 is the same in humans and cows and is not destroyed by pasteurization. In fact, the pasteurization process actually increases IGF-1 levels in milk.

I recommend that you avoid buying milk from cows treated with rBST, if possible. The hormone has become so widely used by dairy farmers that unless the milk label states "from cows not treated with rBST," you should assume that the milk contains the hormone. Most health-food stores sell rBST-free milk. American-made cheeses also contain rBST and excess levels of IGF-1 unless they're labeled "from cows not treated with rBST." Imported European cheeses are safe because Europe has banned rBST.

The good news is that dairy products are not your only possible source of necessary calcium. The foods shown in Table 3-3 are good sources of calcium.

Table 3-3. Calcium Sources: Serving Sizes

Food	Amount	Calcium
Yogurt, plain, low-fat	8 ounces	415
Collards, fresh or frozen, steamed or boiled	1 cup	357
Skim milk	1 cup	306
Spinach, fresh or frozen, steamed or boiled	1 cup	291
Cheese	1 ounce	162
Cottage cheese, 1% milk fat	1 cup	138
Baked beans, canned	1 cup	154
Romaine or red leaf lettuce	1 head	97
Canned salmon	3 ounces	181
Oranges	1 cup	72
Almonds	1 ounce (24 nuts)	70
Black eyed peas, boiled	1 cup	211
Green peas, boiled	1 cup	94

While I recommend that adult women and men consume between 1,200 and 1,500 milligrams (mg) of calcium per day, it is difficult to achieve this goal without supplementation. I will address calcium supplements later in this chapter.

Fruits

✓ EAT 1 SERVING EACH DAY.

Fruits are an important source of fiber, and they are also low in fat and sodium while containing antioxidants and vitamins that contribute to your health. Reach first for color-rich fruits such as blueberries or strawberries.

I recommend the following single serving of fruit each day: half a cup of berries; one medium apple, pear, peach, or banana; or one medium avocado.

Healthy Oils

✓ USE AS NEEDED IN COOKING OR AS A CONDIMENT.

For cooking and salad dressings, you can use extra-virgin olive oil. In addition to providing a delicious flavoring to cooked foods and salads, olive oil has been shown in studies to have a heart-protective benefit. Other healthy oils include canola oil and flaxseed oil. However, because flaxseed oil is heat sensitive, do not use for cooking. Use flaxseed oil for making salad dressings or mixing in yogurt or smoothies.

In contrast, avoid cooking with or consuming margarine, butter, and corn, sunflower, safflower, or peanut oil, as they have been found to promote heart and vascular disease.

Beverages

✓ DRINK EIGHT 8-OUNCE GLASSES EACH DAY.

Very simply, drink water—lots of it, at least eight 8-ounce glasses a day. Drink a glass of water with each meal and then sip throughout the rest of the day. Although water contains no calories and might not contain any micronutrients, it is an indispensable aid to digestion, nutrient absorption, and waste elimination. Add the juice of half a lemon or lime whenever possible; fresh lemon or lime juice relieves symptoms of indigestion such as heartburn, bloating, and belching. Drinking lemon or lime juice regularly aids the bowels in eliminating waste more efficiently, thus controlling constipation and diarrhea. In addition, there is a belief in Ayurvedic medicine (an ancient system of health care native to India) that a cup of hot water with lemon juice in it tones and purifies the liver. Water also impacts how your body metabolizes fat. One of the functions of the liver is to convert stored fat to energy; another is to support kidney function. According to Maia Appleby, author of "Why Drinking Water Really Is the Key to Weight Loss":

> *If the kidneys are water-deprived, the liver has to do their work along with its own, lowering its total productivity. It then can't metabolize fat as quickly or efficiently as it could when the kidneys were pulling their own weight. If you allow this to happen, not only are you being unfair to your liver, but you're also setting yourself up to store fat.*

BELLY-BLASTING DAILY FOOD LIST

Here, for your easy reference, are the recommended foods in their optimum amounts.

Cruciferous vegetables: 2–3 servings a day

Citrus fruits: 1 serving a day

Insoluble fiber: 2 servings a day

Lignans: 2–3 tablespoons a day

Protein: 1 serving with each meal

Calcium: 2 servings a day

Fruit: 1 serving a day (in addition to the citrus)

Healthy Oils: as a condiment

Beverages: eight glasses of water a day

DANGER ZONE: FOODS AND DRINKS THAT INCREASE ESTROGEN LEVELS

Now that you know what foods will decrease your estrogen load and support hormone balance, we want to help you to avoid consuming foods and drinks that can sabotage everything you are doing to lose weight. When it comes to belly fat, the foods and beverages below are the top five spare-tire inflators.

Foods high in saturated fats. These foods have been linked to higher levels of estrogen circulating within the blood. The diet we have recommended therefore excludes the consumption of high-fat meats such as pork sausage, spare ribs, bologna, liverwurst, pork, bacon, ham, frankfurters, and bratwurst, as well as commercial salad dressings, french fries, potato chips, butter, margarine, lard, the shortening in most cookies and pastries, and cream.

Simple carbohydrates. Excessive consumption of refined foods (i.e., the white group) such as sugar, white flour, and white rice has been found to raise blood sugar levels and stimulate insulin release, which then negatively impacts hormone balance. Therefore, this diet does not allow refined or processed foods.

Caffeine. Studies have shown that drinking two cups of coffee a day can increase estrogen levels. In a clinical trial involving approximately 500 women between the ages of thirty-six and forty-five, women who consumed more than one cup of coffee a day had significantly higher levels of estrogen during the early follicular phase of their menstrual cycle. Those who consumed at least 500 mg of caffeine daily, the equivalent of four or five cups of coffee, had nearly 70 percent more estrogen than women who consumed less than 100 mg of caffeine daily. This is why we recommend that you avoid caffeinated products as much as possible, including coffee, caffeinated teas, and caffeinated sodas.

Alcohol. Estrogen is broken down in the liver. If your liver is diseased or overtaxed, it will be unable to efficiently and effectively break down the estrogen circulating in your body. According to the American Liver Association and the American Liver Foundation, liver damage can occur when you consume two drinks a day on a daily basis or five to seven drinks a day on the weekend. Because the liver can heal itself by regenerating damaged tissue, abstinence from alcohol can cause a complete reversal and cure without leaving any residual scarring. How long this will take depends on the degree of liver damage.

Phytoestrogens. Phytoestrogens are naturally occurring estrogenic compounds that are found in a variety of herbs of and spices, such as red clover, black cohosh, chasteberry, and dong quai. Some of the strongest phytoestrogen-containing foods are soy products, including soybeans, soy milk, tofu, tempeh, textured vegetable protein, roasted soybeans, soy granules, miso, and edamame. Although their chemical structure resembles estrogen, it is much less powerful than human estrogen; in fact, its effectiveness is just a thousandth of human estrogen's effectiveness. Unlike lignans, which attach to estrogen and help to reduce estrogen overload through excretion, soy products actually have the potential to compound the problem.

Consumed in moderation, soy products can be healthy food choices for some people. Nevertheless, for the overweight woman or man with a preexisting condition of estrogen dominance, eating too much soy can compound an underlying hormone imbalance. Also, nutritional researchers have identified that in some cases soy products act as a potent antithyroid agent, suppressing thyroid function and causing or worsening hypothyroidism. Because soy products have the potential to be counterproductive to efforts to eliminate estrogen dominance, we recommend eliminating all soy products and other phytoestrogens from your diet. We have found that most people don't miss soy products and can easily find many enjoyable alternatives.

the oops, uh-oh factor: when you just can't say no

Over the years, a number of patients have literally started backing out the door the moment they learned that a hormone-balancing diet required them to avoid all caffeine and alcohol. Although zero consumption of these beverages is ideal for maintaining optimal hormonal balance, if you're one of the women or men who can't imagine your morning without a cup of java or your evening without a toddy, we would not want you to walk away from the plan.

In other words, don't throw out the baby with the bathwater. Do your best. If you don't believe you could possibly give up these beverages, just try to limit your consumption to one cup of coffee in the morning and/or one alcoholic beverage (preferably red wine) in the evening. Although red wine will still tax the liver, research indicates that moderate consumption of red wine might help to protect you from heart disease and can have a positive effect on cholesterol levels and blood pressure.

If you do drink any alcohol, try eating a small fiber-rich snack—such as a piece of fruit or half a cup of whole-grain cereal with skim milk—with a bit of protein, like a bite of chicken or salmon. The food will slow the absorption of the alcohol, so it might help you to avoid a quick buzz and an impulsive order of cheese fries. Then, after one alcoholic drink, order something nonalcoholic and pace yourself.

Finally, if you can't give up your toddies, take milk thistle as a supplement. Medical studies have shown that milk thistle has a protective effect on the liver and will improve its function. We recommend taking a 200 mg milk thistle capsule twice a day.

However, be aware that milk thistle can produce allergic reactions; these tend to be more common among people who are allergic to plants in the same family, such as ragweed, chrysanthemum, marigold, and daisy.

Indulging in these habits will slow down your weight-loss progress a bit, but even small steps will improve your health and your waistline. Ultimately, only you can decide what you are willing to give up in order to lose belly fat.

A MONTH OF HORMONE-BALANCING MEAL PLANS

Instead of obsessing over how many calories you consume, you should focus on eating foods that reduce your estrogen load and support overall hormone balance. Some people like to keep it simple and eat the same foods every day. For instance, a patient named Cynthia has stuck to the meal plan below for nine years.

BREAKFAST: 1 boiled or poached egg, ½ grapefruit, 1 piece of whole-grain toast with ½ teaspoon of all-fruit natural jam, and hot water with the juice of ½ lemon.

LUNCH: 6 ounces of broiled or grilled chicken breast marinated in orange juice and low-sodium soy sauce, steamed broccoli or asparagus, vinegar-marinated coleslaw, and water with lemon.

SNACK: ½ cup of 1% milk fat cottage cheese or 1 cup of plain low-fat yogurt with berries and 2 tablespoons of milled flaxseed.

DINNER: 6 ounces of grilled or broiled fish, spinach salad, steamed cauliflower, brown rice, and water with lemon.

Cynthia continues to be a svelte size 8, so if what works for her works for you, go for it. Most people, however, prefer a bit more variety. As a result, we have developed the following month of sample meal plans. Every day includes tasty new ideas for cooking and serving each of the belly-blasting foods groups. We assure you that if you eat the following three meals a day for a month, you will enjoy each meal, you won't walk around hungry, and you will lose belly fat and inches.

If a dish is followed by an asterisk (*), its recipe can be found in Chapter 8.

DAY 1

BREAKFAST

1 egg scrambled in olive oil. Sprinkle liberally with dill, dried Italian
    seasoning, or 1 tablespoon of fresh salsa, if desired.
1 slice of toasted whole-grain bread; spread with 1 teaspoon of All
    Fruit jam or Smart Balance butter substitute, if desired.
1 small orange
Hot water with the juice of ½ lemon, or herbal tea

LUNCH

Savory Spinach and Salmon Salad*
Grated Beet Salad*
Water with lemon

SNACK

1 medium apple or pear

DINNER

Baked Fish with Basil*
Skillet Broccoli or Asparagus with Sesame Seeds*
Mashed Cauliflower*
Water with lemon

DAY 2

BREAKFAST
½ cup whole-grain or bran cereal with 2 tablespoons ground flaxseed,
    ½ cup fresh berries, and 1 cup skim milk
1 boiled egg
Hot water with juice of ½ lemon, or herbal tea

LUNCH
6 ounnces sliced turkey or chicken breast
Marinated Broccoli, Cucumber, and Tomato Salad*
1 ounce low-fat cheese
Water with lemon

SNACK
¼ cup almonds or ½ cup pumpkin seeds

DINNER
Lentil, Carrot, and Turnip Stew*
Grapefruit and Avocado Salad*
1 slice whole-grain bread
Water with lemon

DAY 3

BREAKFAST
6 ounces broiled or poached salmon, or 1 egg, poached, soft-boiled,
    boiled, or scrambled
Yogurt and Fruit Parfait*
Hot water with juice of ½ lemon, or herbal tea

LUNCH
Veggie Burger*
Best Baked Beans*
Cabbage Apple Salad*
Water with lemon

SNACK
6 celery and carrot sticks
Ginger-Lime Dressing* for dipping

DINNER
6 ounces Rosemary Baked Chicken Breast*
Steamed Brussels sprouts tossed with ground or milled flaxseed
Baked Rutabaga*
Water with lemon

DAY 4

BREAKFAST
Asparagus Omelet*
2 slices turkey bacon
½ cup grapefruit or orange juice
Hot water with juice of ½ lemon, or herbal tea

LUNCH
Not Your Ordinary Tuna Salad*
½ cup marinated cauliflower and cherry tomatoes on a bed of fresh
    spinach
Water with lemon

SNACK
Banana in Bark*

DINNER
Grilled 4-ounce filet of lean beef
½ cup steamed broccoli tossed with sesame seeds
Cruciferous Couscous*
Water with lemon

DAY 5

BREAKFAST
1 poached egg
½ grapefruit
1 slice of toasted whole-grain bread
Hot water with juice of ½ lemon, or herbal tea

LUNCH
Chicken and Asparagus Lettuce Wraps*
1 medium apple or pear
Water with lemon

SNACK
½ cup 1% cottage cheese, mixed with mandarin orange slices and
    2 tablespoons ground or milled flaxseed

DINNER
Grilled Fish with Citrus Marinade*
Simple Greens and Garlic*
½ cup brown rice; may cook in organic chicken, beef, or vegetable
    broth for flavor
Water with lemon

DAY 6

BREAKFAST

½ cup plain low-fat yogurt, mixed with ¼ cup chopped apple and 2 tablespoons ground or milled flaxseed. Add ¼ teaspoon of raw honey and/or cinnamon or nutmeg to taste if desired.

2 slices Canadian or turkey bacon

Hot water with juice of ½ lemon, or herbal tea

LUNCH

Cauliflower and Turkey Bacon Soup*

Simple Cheese Toast*

Water with lemon

SNACK

¼ cup almonds or ½ cup pumpkin seeds

DINNER

Pan-Roasted Fish with Parsley and Bacon*

Skillet Broccoli or Asparagus with Sesame Seeds*

½ cup steamed carrots

Water with lemon

DAY 7

BREAKFAST
½ cup whole-grain or bran cereal with 2 tablespoons ground or milled
    flaxseed, ½ cup fresh berries, and 1 cup skim milk
1 boiled egg
Hot water with juice of ½ lemon, or herbal tea

LUNCH
Favorite Chicken Salad*
Easy Pickled Beets*
Water with lemon

SNACK
1 medium orange or 2 tangerines

DINNER
Quick Turkey-Stuffed Cabbage*
1 ounce low-fat cheese
Water with lemon

DAY 8

BREAKFAST
2 slices turkey bacon
1 slice of toasted whole-grain bread
½ grapefruit
Hot water with juice of ½ lemon, or herbal tea

LUNCH
Spicy Kale and Beans*
1 sliced cucumber and 1 sliced tomato with salt, pepper, Italian season-
    ings, and olive oil or rice wine vinegar
Water with lemon

SNACK
¼ cup almonds or ½ cup pumpkin seeds

DINNER
Lemon Hot Fish*
Grilled Asparagus with Sesame Seeds*
½ cup whole-wheat pasta
Water with lemon

DAY 9

BREAKFAST
Flaxseed and Fruit Smoothie*
6 ounces poached or grilled salmon
Hot water with juice of ½ lemon, or herbal tea

LUNCH
Veggie Burger* Patty (no bun)
Sauerkraut Salad*
1 medium apple or pear
Water with lemon

SNACK
½ cup plain low-fat yogurt, mixed with 1 tablespoon orange juice con-
    centrate, 1 medium orange, and 2 tablespoons ground or milled
    flaxseed

DINNER
6 ounces baked, broiled, or grilled chicken breast; marinate in orange
    juice or fat-free Italian dressing if desired.
Indian-Style Brussels Sprouts*
½ cup steamed yellow squash
1 slice of toasted whole-grain bread; spread with Smart Balance if
    desired.
Water with lemon

DAY 10

BREAKFAST
1 poached or boiled egg
Banana in Bark*
Hot water with juice of ½ lemon, or herbal tea

LUNCH
Chicken and Cold Rice Salad*
Easy Pickled Beets*
Water with lemon

SNACK
1 cup skim milk or 1 cup plain low-fat yogurt (add cinnamon or nut-
    meg if desired) and ½ cup berries with 2 tablespoons ground or
    milled flaxseed

DINNER
Black Beanofritos*
Creamy Coleslaw*
Water with lemon

DAY 11

BREAKFAST
2 slices Canadian or turkey bacon
½ grapefruit
1 slice of toasted whole-grain bread
Hot water with juice of ½ lemon, or herbal tea

LUNCH
6 ounces poached, grilled, or broiled salmon topped with Celebration
    Salsa*
Simple Greens and Garlic*
Water with lemon

SNACK
4–6 carrot and celery sticks with Cucumber and Yogurt Dressing* for
    dipping

DINNER
1 4-ounce ground buffalo or lean sirloin meat patty
Rutabagas and Nutmeg*
Skillet Broccoli or Asparagus with Sesame Seeds*
Water with lemon

DAY 12

BREAKFAST

½ cup plain low-fat yogurt, mixed with ½ cup chopped apple or berries and 2 tablespoons ground or milled flaxseed. Add ¼ teaspoon raw honey and/or cinnamon or nutmeg to taste if desired.

1 egg, boiled, poached, or scrambled; garnish with fresh salsa if desired.

Hot water with juice of ½ lemon, or herbal tea

LUNCH

Tossed Turkey and Spinach Salad*
1 medium orange
Water with lemon

SNACK

¼ cup almonds or ½ cup pumpkin seeds

DINNER

Garlic Chickpeas and Pasta*
½–1 cup sliced cucumber, carrots, and radishes with Cucumber and Yogurt Dressing*
Water with lemon

DAY 13

BREAKFAST
1 poached or boiled egg
Banana in Bark*
Hot water with juice of ½ lemon, or herbal tea

LUNCH
Tuna Melt*
1 medium apple or pear
Water with lemon

SNACK
½ cup 1% cottage cheese, mixed with mandarin orange slices and 2
  tablespoons flaxseed

DINNER
Colorful Turkey Casserole*
Beet and Orange Salad*
1 slice of toasted whole-grain bread
Water with lemon

DAY 14

BREAKFAST
Flaxseed and Fruit Smoothie*
5 ounces poached or grilled salmon
Hot water with juice of ½ lemon, or herbal tea

LUNCH
Turkey, Apple, and Spinach Pita*
Carrot and Orange Salad*
Water with lemon

SNACK
1 medium orange or 2 tangerines

DINNER
Lemon Hot Fish*
Asian Cabbage*
½ cup couscous
Water with lemon

DAY 15

BREAKFAST
Favorite Feta Frittata*
½ cup orange or grapefruit juice
Hot water with juice of ½ lemon, or herbal tea

LUNCH
Orange-Ginger Salmon*
Creamy Coleslaw*
Water with lemon

SNACK
1 cup of berries, tossed with 1 tablespoon plain low-fat yogurt and 2
    tablespoons flaxseed

DINNER
Spicy Kale and Beans*
½ cup brown rice; may cook in organic chicken, beef, or vegetable
    broth for flavor
Water with lemon

DAY 16

BREAKFAST
½ cup whole-grain or bran cereal with 2 tablespoons ground or milled
   flaxseed, ½ cup fresh berries, and 1 cup skim milk
1 link turkey sausage
Hot water with juice of ½ lemon, or herbal tea

LUNCH
6 ounces grilled chicken or turkey breast
Sauerkraut Salad*
1 sliced tomato with salt, pepper, dried Italian seasoning, and olive oil
Water with lemon

SNACK
1 medium apple or pear

DINNER
Fish New Orleans Style*
Beets and Brussels Sprouts*
½ cup brown rice; may cook in organic chicken, beef, or vegetable
   broth for flavor
Water with lemon

DAY 17

BREAKFAST
1 boiled or poached egg
1 medium orange
¼ cup almonds
Hot water with juice of ½ lemon, or herbal tea

LUNCH
5–6 ounces grilled or poached salmon
Cucumber and Yogurt Dressing* as a condiment for the salmon
½ cup steamed asparagus
1 slice of toasted whole-grain bread
Water with lemon

SNACK
Banana in Bark*

DINNER
Garlic Chickpeas and Pasta*
1 cup spinach salad
Water with lemon

DAY 18

BREAKFAST

½ cup plain low-fat yogurt, mixed with ½ cup chopped apple or berries and 2 tablespoons ground or milled flaxseed. Add ½ teaspoon of raw honey and/or cinnamon or nutmeg to taste if desired.
2 slices turkey bacon
Hot water with juice of ½ lemon, or herbal tea

LUNCH

1 cup black beans and ½ cup brown rice
Marinated Cucumber, Radishes, and Onions*
1 whole-wheat tortilla
Water with lemon

SNACK

4–6 celery and carrot sticks
Ginger-Lime Dressing*

DINNER

Cauliflower Crab Cakes*
Skillet Broccoli or Asparagus with Sesame Seeds*
½ cup brown rice; may cook in organic chicken, beef, or vegetable broth for flavor
Water with lemon

DAY 19

BREAKFAST
Asparagus Omelet*
2 slices turkey bacon
½ cup grapefruit or orange juice
Hot water with juice of ½ lemon, or herbal tea

LUNCH
Favorite Chicken Salad* on bed of fresh spinach
Carrot and Orange Salad*
Water with lemon

SNACK
1 cup of berries, tossed with 1 tablespoon plain low-fat yogurt and 2
    tablespoons flaxseed

DINNER
Nest of Beans and Greens*
Simple Cheese Toast*
Water with lemon

DAY 20

BREAKFAST
½ cup whole-grain or bran cereal, with 2 tablespoons ground or milled
    flaxseed, ½ cup fresh berries, and 1 cup skim milk
1 boiled egg
Hot water with juice of ½ lemon, or herbal tea

LUNCH
Open-Faced Veggie Cheeseburger*
Marinated Cucumber, Radishes, and Onions*
Water with lemon

SNACK
1 medium orange or 2 tangerines

DINNER
Baked Fish with Basil*
Broccoli and Cauliflower in Lime Dressing*
½ cup cooked Carrots; may season with dill, Italian seasoning, or a
    spray of Smart Balance if desired.
Water with lemon

DAY 21

BREAKFAST
1 poached egg
½ grapefruit
1 slice of toasted whole-grain bread
Hot water with juice of ½ lemon, or herbal tea

LUNCH
Turkey and Asparagus Wrap*
1 medium apple or pear
Water with lemon

PARTY!
Celebration! In three weeks, you've probably lost 7–10 pounds. Instead of having your everyday snack, have a party. Invite your friends over and let them in on your secret. Serve the following:
Marinated vegetable potpourri
Simple Cheese Toast*
Spinach dip and raw vegetables
Sparkling water with a splash of cranberry or orange juice served in champagne glasses; drop in a few raspberries for color and zing. (Make sure the cranberry juice is 100% fruit juice and not the kind that is sweetened with high-fructose corn syrup.)

DINNER
6 ounces grilled Salmon with Dill and Lemon*
½ cup spinach salad
½ cup brown rice; may cook in organic chicken, beef, or vegetable broth for flavor
Water with lemon

DAY 22

BREAKFAST

1 egg, scrambled in olive oil. Sprinkle liberally with dill or dried Italian seasoning if desired.

1 slice of toasted whole-grain bread; spread with Smart Balance if desired.

1 small orange

Hot water with juice of ½ lemon, or herbal tea

LUNCH

Savory Spinach and Salmon Salad*

Cabbage-Apple Salad*

Water with lemon

SNACK

1 medium orange or 2 tangerines

DINNER

Baked Fish with Basil*

Skillet Broccoli or Asparagus with Sesame Seeds*

Mashed Cauliflower*

Water with lemon

DAY 23

BREAKFAST
½ cup whole-grain or bran cereal with 2 tablespoons ground or milled
   flaxseed, ½ cup berries, and 1 cup skim milk
1 boiled egg
Hot water with juice of ½ lemon, or herbal tea

LUNCH
6 ounces sliced turkey or chicken breast
Spinach Salad with Beets in Cottage Cheese*
Water with lemon

SNACK
¼ cup almonds or ½ cup pumpkin seeds

DINNER
Spicy Kale and Beans*
1 medium apple or pear
1 slice whole-grain bread
Water with lemon

DAY 24

BREAKFAST
4–6 ounces broiled or poached salmon
Yogurt and Fruit Parfait*
Hot water with juice of ½ lemon, or herbal tea

LUNCH
Veggie Burger*
Best Baked Beans*
Cabbage and Apple Salad*
Water with lemon

SNACK
4–6 celery and carrot sticks
Ginger-Lime Dressing* for dipping

DINNER
Rosemary Baked Chicken Breast*
Green and Yellow Veggie Hash*
½ cup Brown rice
Water with lemon

DAY 25

BREAKFAST
Asparagus Omelet*
2 slices turkey bacon
¾ cup grapefruit or orange juice
Hot water with juice of ½ lemon, or herbal tea

LUNCH
Not Your Ordinary Tuna Salad*
Water with lemon
Rutabagas and Nutmeg*

SNACK
Banana in Bark*

DINNER
Grilled 4-ounce filet of lean beef
Cruciferous Couscous*
Roasted Beets*
Water with lemon

DAY 26

BREAKFAST
1 poached egg
½ grapefruit
1 slice of toasted whole-grain bread; spread with 1 teaspoon of All
     Fruit jam or Smart Balance if desired
Hot water with juice of ½ lemon, or herbal tea

LUNCH
1 turkey hot dog, grilled
Kale and Sauerkraut*
1 sliced tomato; drizzle with olive oil and balsamic vinegar if desired.
Water with lemon

SNACK
½ cup 1% cottage cheese, mixed with mandarin orange slices and 2
     tablespoons ground or milled flaxseed

DINNER
Grilled Fish with Citrus Marinade*
Simple Greens and Garlic*
Spinach and Feta Brown Rice*
Water with lemon

DAY 27

BREAKFAST
½ cup plain low-fat yogurt, mixed with ¼ cup chopped apple and 2
tablespoons ground or milled flaxseed. Add ¼ teaspoon of raw
honey and/or cinnamon or nutmeg to taste if desired.
2 slices turkey bacon
Hot water with juice of ½ lemon, or herbal tea

LUNCH
Cauliflower and Turkey Bacon Soup*
Simple Cheese Toast*
Water with lemon

SNACK
¼ cup almonds or ½ cup pumpkin seeds

DINNER
6 ounces grilled fish (drizzle with lemon or marinade with lemon juice
or salsa)
Lemon-Curry Cauliflower and Kale*
½ cup steamed carrots seasoned with salt, pepper, and dried dill if
desired
Water with lemon

DAY 28

BREAKFAST

½ cup whole-grain or bran cereal, with 2 tablespoons ground or milled flaxseed, ½ cup fresh berries, and 1 cup skim milk

1 boiled egg

Hot water with juice of ½ lemon, or herbal tea

LUNCH

Favorite Chicken Salad*

Beet and Orange Salad*

Water with lemon

SNACK

1 medium orange or 2 tangerines

DINNER

Baked Fish with Basil*

Dressed-Up Asparagus*

½ cup brown rice; may cook in organic chicken, beef, or vegetable broth for flavor

Water with lemon

DAY 29

BREAKFAST
2 slices turkey bacon
1 slice of toasted whole-grain bread; spread with 1 teaspoon All Fruit jam or Smart Balance if desired.
½ grapefruit
Hot water with juice of ½ lemon, or herbal tea

LUNCH
Spicy Kale and Beans*
1 sliced cucumber and 1 sliced tomato; may dress with low-fat balsamic vinegar dressing
Water with lemon

SNACK
¼ cup almonds or ½ cup pumpkin seeds

DINNER
Lemon Hot Fish*
½ cup steamed broccoli tossed with olive oil and garlic
½ cup whole-wheat pasta, mixed with diced tomato, olive oil, and fresh basil
Water with lemon

DAY 30

BREAKFAST
Flaxseed and Fruit Smoothie*
4–6 ounces poached or grilled salmon
Hot water with juice of ½ lemon, or herbal tea

LUNCH
Veggie Burger* Patty (no bun)
Sauerkraut Salad*
Sliced apple
Water with lemon

SNACK
½ cup plain low-fat yogurt, mixed with 1 tablespoon orange juice concentrate, 1 medium orange, and 2 tablespoons ground or milled flaxseed.

DINNER
6 ounces baked, broiled, or grilled chicken breast
Indian-Style Brussels Sprouts*
½ cup steamed yellow squash
1 slice of toasted whole-grain bread; spread with 1 teaspoon Smart Balance if desired.
Water with lemon

Sticking to this nutritional plan will go a long way toward balancing your hormones and will help you lose weight; however, for those wanting to get rid of estrogen dominance and belly fat quickly and for good, there are two more important steps you have to take. The next two chapters will tell you exactly what they are.

STEP 2:
USE PROGESTERONE—THE
SIMPLE WAY TO A FLAT BELLY

A lthough the title of this chapter might sound too good to be true, the success of thousands of patients has shown this to be a reality. By boosting your body's progesterone levels, you can take an important step toward correcting your underlying condition of estrogen dominance and finally lose those pounds. You will also make a large stride in improving your overall health and well-being.

how to safely and effectively boost declining progesterone levels

If your progesterone production has declined and you are estrogen dominant, then common sense would indicate that in order to reestablish hormonal equilibrium, you have to add progesterone back into your body. The theory is very simple, but unfortunately there is a great deal of confusion about hormone replacement therapies.

Over the last several years, hormone replacement has frequently been in the news. In magazine articles and on television shows, celebrities have bandied around terms like *natural, bio-identical, synthetic,* and *pharmaceutical* as if they were interchangeable. They are not.

Natural human hormones are produced within your body by the ovaries or testes, the adrenal glands, and the hypothalamus. These hormones travel through the bloodstream to fit into specific hormone receptor sites located throughout your body and brain. Each hormone receptor site will recognize the specific molecular structure of only a single type of hormone. This means that a receptor site for progesterone will not recognize estrogen or testosterone; it will recognize only the molecular structure of progesterone.

Natural human hormones attach to their receptor sites like keys fitting into locks. The chemical term for this key-and-lock phenomenon is *relative binding affinity* (RBA). Natural human hormones have a 100 percent RBA for their respective receptor sites.

what every woman needs to know: the danger of synthetic hormones

Bio-identical hormones are derived from plants, usually soybeans or wild yams. This biochemical process ensures that the molecular structure of bio-identical hormones is identical to that of the natural human hormones produced in the body. When introduced into the body, bio-identical hormones *fit perfectly* into the hormone receptor lock and trigger exactly the same response as the one previously fostered by the hormones produced in the ovaries or testes, the adrenal gland, and the hypothalamus.

Bio-identical hormones also have a 100 percent RBA for the hormone receptor sites within the body. Because the body recognizes and accepts bio-identical hormones just as it would recognize and accept naturally occurring human hormones, bio-identical hormone replacement is both safe and effective.

The molecular structure of natural human hormones cannot be patented; thus, neither can the identical molecular structure of bio-identical hormones. Without a patent, how could pharmaceutical companies protect their formulations and, most important, their profits? The answer is that they can't. Consequently, for almost three-quarters of a century, pharmaceutical companies have been developing, patenting, and marketing hormones that have a slightly different molecular structure from natural human hormones and bio-identical hormones. The pharmaceutically produced and patented hormones are correctly referred to as synthetic hormones. The list of synthetic hormones on the market today includes such brand names as Premarin, Prempro, Menest, Ortho-est, Activella, and Femhrt. There are many others.

Synthetic hormones have shapes that are not found in nature. They fit poorly with the body's hormone receptors and therefore produce unnatural chemical reactions and striking alterations in biological activity. Their RBA is often much less than 100 percent, which results in side effects and health risks. Premarin, for instance, is metabolized horse estrogen with a low affinity for binding with any human hormone receptor. Premarin is also 49.3 percent estrone (E1), the cancer-promoting estrogen. This is almost ten times the percentage that occurs naturally within the body.

Many medical studies have substantiated the dangers of synthetic hormone replacement. In July 2002, the National Institutes of Health (NIH) halted a large study examining the effects of a widely used synthetic hormone, Prempro, which combines the altered molecular structures for both estrogen and progesterone. The study, which was one of five major studies in a large clinical trial called the Women's Health Initiative, was discontinued because the synthetic hormones were found to increase a woman's risk of breast cancer as well as heart disease, blood clots, and stroke. Later findings also linked synthetic hormone replacement to an increased risk for Alzheimer's disease. The findings were published in *The Journal of the American Medical Association.*

Unfortunately, bio-identical progesterone is often confused with synthetically produced progestin. The Women's Health Initiative used progestin, *not* bio-identical progesterone. There is no documented evidence in the scientific literature of any cases of cancer resulting from treatment with bio-identical progesterone.

In contrast, studies reported in both the International Society for Preventive Oncology's *Cancer Detection and Prevention Journal* (1999) and the International Union Against Cancer's *International Cancer Journal* (2005) found that women who used synthetic progestins plus estrogen had a significantly higher risk of breast cancer, whereas women using bio-identical progesterone plus synthetic estrogens had a lower risk of breast cancer than women using estrogen alone.

READER/CUSTOMER CARE SURVEY

We care about your opinions! Please take a moment to fill out our online Reader Survey at **http://survey.hcibooks.com**.

As a **"THANK YOU"** you will receive a **VALUABLE INSTANT COUPON** towards future book purchases

as well as a **SPECIAL GIFT** available only online! Or, you may mail this card back to us.

(PLEASE PRINT IN ALL CAPS)

First Name _____ MI. _____ Last Name _____

Address _____ City _____

State _____ Zip _____ Email _____

1. Gender
- ☐ Female
- ☐ Male

2. Age
- ☐ 8 or younger
- ☐ 9-12
- ☐ 13-16
- ☐ 17-20
- ☐ 21-30
- ☐ 31+

3. Did you receive this book as a gift?
- ☐ Yes
- ☐ No

4. Annual Household Income
- ☐ under $25,000
- ☐ $25,000 - $34,999
- ☐ $35,000 - $49,999
- ☐ $50,000 - $74,999
- ☐ over $75,000

5. What are the ages of the children living in your house?
- ☐ 0 - 14
- ☐ 15+

6. Marital Status
- ☐ Single
- ☐ Married
- ☐ Divorced
- ☐ Widowed

7. How did you find out about the book?
(please choose one)
- ☐ Recommendation
- ☐ Store Display
- ☐ Online
- ☐ Catalog/Mailing
- ☐ Interview/Review

8. Where do you usually buy books?
(please choose one)
- ☐ Bookstore
- ☐ Online
- ☐ Book Club/Mail Order
- ☐ Price Club (Sam's Club, Costco's, etc.)
- ☐ Retail Store (Target, Wal-Mart, etc.)

9. What subject do you enjoy reading about the most?
(please choose one)
- ☐ Parenting/Family
- ☐ Relationships
- ☐ Recovery/Addictions
- ☐ Health/Nutrition
- ☐ Christianity
- ☐ Spirituality/Inspiration
- ☐ Business Self-help
- ☐ Women's Issues
- ☐ Sports

10. What attracts you most to a book?
(please choose one)
- ☐ Title
- ☐ Cover Design
- ☐ Author
- ☐ Content

Health Communications, Inc.
3201 SW 15th Street
Deerfield Beach FL 33442-9875

FOLD HERE

Comments

marketing a dangerous lie

If bio-identical hormone replacement is so safe, you might be wondering why so many physicians continue to prescribe synthetic hormones. The answer is a combination of ignorance, confusion, and marketing. Pharmaceutical companies make billions of dollars selling synthetic hormone products. In terms of the safety of synthetic versus bio-identical hormone replacement, pharmaceutical companies have a lot to lose. Consequently, these companies spend millions of dollars marketing synthetic hormones to physicians by sponsoring continuing medical education (CME) programs, office lunch presentations, and off-site forums at resort locations.

In her book, *The Truth About the Drug Companies*, Dr. Marcia Angell, former editor in chief of *The New England Journal of Medicine*, states: "Drug companies have become vast marketing machines wielding nearly limitless influence over medical research, education and how doctors do their jobs."

There are volumes of solid, credible clinical trials and medical studies that validate the safety and efficacy of bio-identical hormone therapies. Unfortunately, the medical research institutions and universities that publish these studies do not have the budget to hire a sales force to go out into the field to educate physicians. Consequently, most doctors continue to remain unenlightened regarding the science behind the safe treatment option of bio-identical hormones.

how bio-identical progesterone kick-starts weight loss at a cellular level

Bio-identical progesterone neutralizes estrogen dominance, thereby kick-starting weight loss at a cellular level. Here's what happens.

First, progesterone eliminates the hypothyroid condition. Estrogen causes food calories to be stored as fat; the thyroid hormone causes fat calories to be turned into usable energy. Estrogen and the thyroid hormone therefore have opposing actions. Estrogen dominance inhibits thyroid action and lowers the rate of metabolism of the body. Progesterone inhibits estrogen action, thereby allowing the thyroid hormone to function properly. In other words, progesterone triggers a metabolic response that allows weight loss to occur.

Second, when progesterone is added back into the body, it acts as a natural diuretic, which helps to reduce bloating.

Finally, when progesterone and estrogen levels are rebalanced, the rapid release of insulin is tempered. The result is normalized blood sugar levels and reduced food cravings.

the health benefits of bio-identical progesterone

In addition to helping with weight loss, bio-identical progesterone brings numerous health benefits.

protection from cancer

As previously described, estrogen increases cell growth, and when unchecked, this cell growth can result in cancer. In

contrast, bio-identical progesterone replacement can neutral-
ize or reduce estrogen's ability to stimulate cell growth.
According to several medical studies, when internal progesterone levels are boosted to balance estrogen levels, there is
not enough extra estrogen circulating within the body to
stimulate estrogen receptor-positive tumor growth.

Dr. Uzzi Reiss, founder of the Beverly Hills Anti-Aging
Center and coauthor of *Natural Hormone Balance for Women*,
explains as follows:

> *Progesterone is the most protective breast hormone. At an
> infertility clinic at Johns Hopkins, Linda Cowan published a
> study in the early 1980s. She followed two groups of women
> for more than 20 years. There aren't many studies like this.
> What's unique about these women is that one group had
> blocked fallopian tubes, and the other group had progesterone
> deficiency. The only long-term health effect the women with
> blocked tubes had was the inability to get pregnant. But more
> than 20 years later, the group with progesterone deficiency had
> tenfold more cancer.*

How could this be? It's very simple: progesterone functions to inhibit cells from replicating. Progesterone increases
the activity of a gene called P53, which protects us from cancer. It also down-regulates and decreases the function of
BCL2, a gene that is a marker for cancer.

The role of hormone balance in the development and prevention of hormone-dependent cancers is still a subject of
much controversy in the conventional medical community.
More research is definitely needed in this area; however, in

more than a decade of treating thousands of women suffering from hormone imbalances, I have only had two patients who were later diagnosed with breast cancer. This is far below the national average. According to statistics from the American Cancer Society, the chance of an American woman developing invasive breast cancer at some time in her life is about one in eight; that's 12.5 percent of all American women. Wouldn't it be nice if someday we would read about a scientific study that tracked a huge reduction in breast cancer rates because every woman in the United States augmented her body's progesterone level as soon as her hormone levels began to shift?

cardiac health

Bio-identical progesterone replacement is also good for heart health. Because heart disease is the number one killer of women in America, the effect of progesterone on cardiac health has been an area of extensive research. You will recall that the Women's Health Initiative trial indicated that synthetic estrogen plus progestin increased cardiac risk. The good news is that researchers have proven that a hormone replacement regimen consisting of both bio-identical estrogen and bio-identical progesterone serves to reduce coronary vascular activity. In other words, whether progesterone is produced within the body naturally or is a bio-identical formulation added back into the body, it definitively balances estrogen and has a cardioprotective effect.

osteoporosis prevention

Progesterone is also responsible for the stimulation of bone building that can prevent or treat osteoporosis. Dr. Morris Noteloviz, author of *Estrogen, Yes or No?* states, "Progesterone receptors are present in osteoblasts. Based on *in vivo* (in the body) and clinical studies, it is now believed that bio-identical progesterone replacement may stimulate new bone formation, although the mechanism has not yet been identified."

A 1996 study published in *The Journal of the American Medical Association* found that women using bio-identical progesterone cream experienced an average of 7 to 8 percent bone mineral density increase in the first year, 4 to 5 percent in the second year, and 3 to 4 percent in the third year. Untreated women in this category typically lose 1.5 percent bone mineral density per year. For the treatment and prevention of bone density loss, no other form of hormone replacement or dietary supplementation has had as high a level of positive response as bio-identical progesterone.

PMS relief

Have you or anyone you know ever suffered from premenstrual syndrome (PMS)? If so, here is more good news about progesterone. In the early 1950s, a theory was advanced within the medical community that PMS was caused by unopposed estrogen during the luteal phase of your menstrual cycle. The luteal phase is the time period beginning with the day after ovulation and running through the remainder of your menstrual cycle (it ends the day before your next period). Typically, the duration of the luteal phase lasts between ten and sixteen days, and is generally consistent from cycle to cycle, averaging for most women at fourteen days. To test this theory, researchers administered bio-identical progesterone by intramuscular injection, vaginal or rectal suppository, or subcutaneous pellets. Bio-identical progesterone resolved PMS symptoms in 83 percent of the women in the study.

improved memory and moods

Estrogen and progesterone must be in balance for the brain to function properly. Estrogen increases brain stimulation and fosters clear thinking and good memory. Progesterone is very important to the central nervous system; it has been proven to promote healthy sleep patterns and a sense of calm. Progesterone is often referred to as the "feel-good" hormone. Although progesterone's effect on mood and sense of well-being is very relevant, there is also new evidence that it might play an even more critical role in long-term mental functioning. Recent research has shown that an imbalance in estrogen and progesterone levels could be a precursor to Alzheimer's disease.

improved quality of life

Medical research studies provide clear physiological and biochemical evidence of the many health benefits of bio-identical progesterone replacement. For instance, the Mayo Clinic published a study in the *Journal of Women's Health* in

2000 that showed that women who included bio-identical progesterone in their hormone replacement regimen were more satisfied with their overall quality of life. The study participants also reported that they felt an improvement in several other health areas, including relief of sleep disturbances, hot flashes, anxiety, and symptoms of depression.

forms of bio-identical progesterone

Bio-identical progesterone can be administered as a cream, a pill, a capsule, a gelcap, drops under the tongue, or a suppository. Fortunately, for those who don't like taking pills, topical creams have been shown to be the most effective way of administering bio-identical progesterone. If you take bio-identical progesterone in a pill, it must first go through the liver to be metabolized. Some of the active substance is automatically excreted in the feces. The remaining progesterone must be metabolized into more than thirty-five biochemical substances before it can enter the bloodstream. This means that only a fraction of the progesterone contained in the pill makes its way into your bloodstream. When applied to your skin, however, the progesterone goes directly into your bloodstream. Once it is in your bloodstream, all of the progesterone in the cream travels to the progesterone receptor sites and is utilized by progesterone target tissues. Very simply, bio-identical progesterone cream allows the body to recognize and use the bio-identical hormone replacement in exactly the same way it would use progesterone produced by the ovaries. Furthermore, the body's response to the cream is more immediate with a lower dosage.

HOW TO USE PROGESTERONE ON THE PLAN

To use bio-identical progesterone, follow these guidelines:

- If you're a woman who is still menstruating regularly, apply the cream twice daily from days 8 to 26 of your cycle. In other words, *do not apply when menstruating*.
- If you're a woman who is no longer menstruating due to menopause or a hysterectomy, who is peri-menopausal, or who is having irregular periods, apply the cream twice daily for twenty-five days. Then take five days off. (You may begin using the cream on any day you choose.)
- If you're a woman who is also on a regimen of bio-identical estrogen, you should apply bio-identical progesterone cream twice daily, every day. (Bio-identical estrogen replacement will be discussed later.)
- If you're a man older than forty, you should also apply the cream twice daily for twenty-five days. Then take five days off. (You may begin using the cream on any day you choose.)

Bio-identical progesterone cream is readily available without a prescription. You can purchase formulations at compounding pharmacies with a physician's prescription or over the counter at most health food stores and some natural product websites.

Here is the bad news: some over-the-counter progesterone creams are better than others. The reason for this discrepancy is that there is no regulatory body that oversees the production or standardization of manufacturing so-called natural products. This means that there is great variation among the many over-the-counter progesterone creams on the market today.

I stumbled onto the discrepancy ten years ago when I first began treating patients. Determining from their symptoms that my patients needed bio-identical progesterone replacement, I would recommend that they purchase an over-the-counter progesterone cream and apply it twice a day, yet I didn't direct them to any specific brand. I would then ask them to return in six weeks so I could monitor their response and symptom improvement.

After six weeks, some patients reported great improvement—or even elimination of—their symptoms. Others reported less than satisfying results. The discrepancy led me to think that certain products were more helpful than others. Drawing on my pharmacological background, I did some research to determine which formulations work the best and why.

what to look for in a progesterone cream

The ideal progesterone cream is a bio-identical formulation of progesterone and not just a mixture of natural remedies for hormone replacement. The confusion between the two is caused by the fact that the parent molecule for progesterone comes from a substance known as diosgenin, which is found in soy and in Mexican wild yam. Many products on the market today that contain soy or Mexican wild yam claim to be natural progesterone; however, they won't work in the body in the same way that bio-identical progesterone does. Until the diosgenin molecule is converted in a laboratory from its original molecular structure to that of bio-identical progesterone, the body will not recognize it. Consequently, soy or Mexican wild yam in a raw state will not effectively impact the underlying hormonal imbalance or its symptoms.

For the best and purest product on the market, the bio-identical progesterone used in the cream must meet the U.S. Pharmacopoeia gold standard for quality. This should be clearly marked on the product label.

In addition, the lab in which the bio-identical progesterone is compounded should operate under the strict guidelines of the National Association of Compounding Pharmacists. This is not required by law, so not all product manufacturers go to the trouble or expense.

The progesterone molecule in the cream should be designed to be released over time. This is critical, because if the cream is immediately absorbed through the skin, it will result in a quick spike in progesterone levels and a temporary rather than constant relief of symptoms. The importance of a time-controlled delivery system is that optimal hormonal balance is restored continuously so that users of the cream experience continuous relief of their symptoms throughout the day. The term *liposomal formulation* or *liposomal delivery* should be clearly visible on the product label.

In our first book, *From Hormone Hell to Hormone Well*, we include a list of several over-the-counter bio-identical progesterone creams that we have personally analyzed and have found to meet the above criteria. You can also find information about my personal formulation of bio-identical progesterone cream on my website www.hormonewell.com.

Prior to his death in 2003, Dr. John R. Lee, the primary author of the *What Your Doctor May Not Tell You About Menopause* series and a recognized pioneer in the field of bio-identical hormone replacement, worked with coauthor Virginia Hopkins to provide a list of reviewed and approved over-the-counter progesterone creams. You can find his original listing in the back of his books. Today, Ms. Hopkins continues Dr. Lee's mission by regularly updating his original list of preferred creams on his website (www. johnleemd.com/store/resource_progesteronc.html).

Remember estrogen-dominant Evelyn and Richard from Chapter 2? Although they were both skeptical that simply rubbing on a cream twice a day would have any real benefit, they agreed to give it a try. Just six weeks later Evelyn called to report the following:

> *Dr. Randolph, I honestly didn't hold much stock in what you told me, but because I felt desperate, I was willing to give anything a try. Within three weeks of using your progesterone cream, my stomach felt less bloated, and I weighed six pounds less. I also found that I felt calmer throughout the day, and at night I slept without waking for the first time in years.*
>
> *Richard has actually lost eight pounds in just six weeks. Soon after he started using your cream, he began to act more like his old self. He started coming home, and instead of plopping down on the sofa with a beer, he would take a thirty- to forty-minute walk. He has also begun to have more energy in our bedroom, if you know what I mean. We both feel like your progesterone cream is a miracle potion.*

Bio-identical progesterone replacement is no miracle potion, but when you restore the hormone that your body is missing, the results will often feel miraculous. Because boosting your deficient progesterone level is a critical first step in neutralizing an underlying condition of estrogen dominance, don't wait until you've finished this book to get started. The sooner you begin using bio-identical progesterone cream, the better chance you have of making quick progress toward your weight-loss and waist-size goals.

STEP 3:
TAKE THE RIGHT SUPPLEMENTS
TO SUPPORT, NOT SABOTAGE,
YOUR HORMONE BALANCE

(5)

Over the last several years, I have researched and tested hordes of nutritional supplements. My goal has been to identify those supplements that could positively influence estrogen metabolism. I have found a select group of supplements that will enhance healthy hormone balance and thus promote weight loss and weight management. These are described below.

Calcium D-Glucarate

Calcium D-glucarate is a natural substance that promotes the body's detoxification process and supports hormonal balance. Calcium D-glucarate facilitates the detoxification process by inhibiting the reabsorption of estrogen-like toxins into the bloodstream, allowing them to leave the body and be excreted in the feces.

Calcium D-glucarate has been found to lower unhealthy estrogen levels in animals and thereby inhibit the development or progression of cancer.

✓ TAKE 1,000 MG OF CALCIUM D-GLUCARATE TWICE DAILY.

Diindolylmethane (DIM)

Diindolylmethane (DIM) is a phytonutrient akin to the indole-3-carbinol (I3C) found in cruciferous vegetables. DIM has unique hormonal benefits. It supports the activity of enzymes that improve estrogen metabolism by increasing the levels of 2-hydroxyestrone—that is, the good estrogen. When taken as part of a healthy diet, DIM helps to relieve PMS symptoms and to promote fat loss and healthy estrogen metabolism.

In men, DIM also promotes its own metabolism. This means that it allows for greater testosterone activity. Men who take DIM supplements will benefit biochemically because DIM promotes an optimal testosterone-to-estrogen ratio.

✓ WOMEN SHOULD TAKE 200 MG OF DIM PER DAY; MEN SHOULD TAKE 400 MG PER DAY.

The B Vitamins

The B vitamins—B_1, B_2, B_3, B_5, B_6, B_{12}, and folate—do a lot within your body to support estrogen detoxification.

Conversely, if your body is deficient in B vitamins, you will have higher levels of circulating estrogen. By now, you definitely know that increased estrogen levels lead to estrogen dominance—and estrogen dominance will most certainly lead to weight gain and the inability to get rid of that weight.

B vitamins also impact estrogen activity for the hormone receptors at the cellular level. Clinical studies have shown that high levels of intracellular (i.e., within the cell) B_6 can decrease the binding response at the estrogen hormone receptor site. What happens at the cellular level is sort of like an internal game of musical chairs: if the music stops and B_6 sits down in the "estrogen chair," then the estrogen molecule is out of the game.

✓ BECAUSE THE B VITAMINS WORK TOGETHER TO PERFORM SUCH VITAL TASKS AT THE CELLULAR LEVEL, YOU SHOULD TAKE A B-COMPLEX VITAMIN, NOT JUST ONE OR TWO OF THE B VITAMINS. Take a B-complex that has 50–100 mg each of thiamine (B_1), riboflavin (B_2), niacin (B_3), pantothenic acid (B_5), and B_6 (a water-soluble vitamin that exists in three major chemical forms: pyridoxine, pyridoxal, and pyridoxamine), along with PABA, choline, inositol, 50 micrograms (mcg) of B_{12}, and 400 mcg of folic acid.

Vitamin E

Years ago, researchers studied the effects of vitamin E in reducing the difficulties of menopause, and most of these studies found vitamin E to be helpful. Vitamin E has also been shown to reduce PMS-related breast tenderness, nervousness, depression, headache, fatigue, and insomnia. Newer research suggests that low vitamin E levels are linked to estrogen dominance. Furthermore, vitamin E deficiency has been found to inhibit estrogen detoxification.

✓ TAKE 400 IU OF VITAMIN E PER DAY.

Calcium-Magnesium Combo

Most women and men find it difficult to get the recommended 1,200–1,500 mg of calcium per day from their diet. Calcium intake should therefore be supplemented with a calcium-magnesium combination supplement. The right kind of fat is necessary for calcium availability in the soft tissues and to promote calcium elevation in the bloodstream so that muscles contract properly and maintain their tone, nerves function smoothly, blood clots when needed, and bones and teeth remain strong and healthy. Women who believe they are getting enough calcium through diet and supplements may be sabotaging themselves if they do not include enough of the right oils (i.e. extra-virgin olive, canola, or flaxseed oils) in their diets. Also, because this diet includes minimum animal products and sodium and little or no sugar or caffeine, your body should better retain its nutritional and supplemental calcium.

Magnesium is another element that helps the body to eliminate excess estrogen. For women, magnesium levels tend to fall at certain times during the menstrual cycle. These shifts in magnesium levels can upset an optimal calcium-magnesium ratio. When the two minerals are in proper balance, the body better absorbs and assimilates the calcium it needs and also allows calcium to migrate from tissue and organs where it doesn't belong.

Without magnesium, calcium might not be fully utilized. Underabsorption of calcium can lead to menstrual cramps. As with a vitamin E deficiency, when the body does not have enough magnesium to support calcium absorption, many women report PMS symptoms such as mood swings, fatigue, headaches, and sleeplessness.

Premenstrual chocolate craving is a phenomenon that has puzzled many physicians. They have been unable to explain why some women have this overwhelming urge to eat lots of chocolate right before their periods, yet at other times of the month the women's chocolate cravings are not as strong. The PMS-chocolate connection makes a lot of sense because chocolate is very high in magnesium.

Keeping a balance of calcium and magnesium is critical for optimal physical functioning and for hormone balance.

✓ YOU SHOULD TAKE A CALCIUM-MAGNESIUM SUPPLEMENT THAT CONTAINS A RATIO OF TWO PARTS CALCIUM (1,500 MG) TO ONE PART MAGNESIUM (750 MG).

7-Keto Dehydroepiandrosterone (DHEA)

Dehydroepiandrosterone (DHEA) is one of the hormones produced by the adrenal glands. After being secreted by the adrenal glands, DHEA circulates in the bloodstream as DHEA-sulfate (DHEAS) and is converted, as needed, into other hormones. Since it is a precursor to testosterone, DHEA may help to build muscle. It is very unusual for anyone under the age of thirty-five or forty to have low DHEA levels. As we age, however, the body's production of DHEA declines, so people older than forty can most definitely become DHEA-deficient.

Although many anti-aging enthusiasts are familiar with DHEA, far fewer are likely to be aware of its metabolite, 7-keto DHEA, which within the body to safely boost immune function and help reduce body fat. The term *7-keto DHEA* is in fact a brand name for the chemical compound 3-acetyl-7-dehydroepiandrosterone. Human blood levels of both DHEA and 7-keto DHEA tend to rise and fall in a similar pattern with age: increasing until the twenties, beginning to decline in the thirties, and continuing to decline until the levels are reduced by about 50 percent by age fifty. Clinical studies have shown that as 7-keto DHEA levels go down in middle age, body weight tends to goes up.

Weight loss is stimulated by 7-keto DHEA through a process called *thermogenesis*, the creation of heat at a cellular level. The more thermogenesis, the higher the metabolic rate and the more that fat is literally burned up as energy. Studies have also demonstrated that 7-keto DHEA does not accumulate in the body over time and that it is free of unhealthy side effects.

Supplementation with 7-keto DHEA is significantly beneficial for increasing the rate at which the body converts stored fat into energy. Because 7-keto DHEA is a natural hormone metabolite, it benefits the body in two ways: it helps to restore hormone balance while also working internally to melt away those unwanted pounds.

✓ TAKE 100 MG OF 7-KETO DHEA PER DAY, ONE CAPSULE EVERY MORNING.

Chitosan

Chitosan, which is processed from the shells of crustaceans such as shrimp, lobster, and crab, acts as a super fiber. Its swelling action creates a sensation of feeling full, thereby serving to suppress the appetite. In addition, the super-fiber characteristics of chitosan foster a natural cleansing process that is vital to weight loss.

Chitosan is also able to absorb six to ten times its weight in fat and oils. It then converts the fat molecules into a form that the human body does not absorb. Because chitosan causes less fat to enter the body, the body has to turn to previously stored body fat to burn for energy. The net result is weight loss.

✓ TAKE 750 MG TO 1 GRAM (G) OF CHITOSAN THREE TIMES A DAY WITH MEALS.

PART 3

KEEPING THAT *flat* BELLY FOR LIFE

Are you concerned about putting the three steps—diet, proges-terone, and supplements—into an easy framework that you can use every day? This section shows you how to integrate these steps into your daily life and how to make hormone-healthy choices that support your weight-loss goals.

A fear of rebound weight gain is common in people who follow this three-step plan and finally take off those extra pounds around their middle. The good news is that these fears almost always prove to be unfounded. Years go by and people on this plan delightedly maintain their desired weight and waistlines.

Why does this plan work for life when other diets have short bursts of weight loss followed by permanent rebound weight gain? Because it is much more than a diet; it is a positive, healthy life plan. Stress and poor lifestyle choices can sabotage your hormone balance and thus your long-term weight loss.

This section provides a simple framework you can put into action every day to keep your weight off for the long term. We tell you how to make hormone-healthy choices in four key areas that affect your hormones and your weight: managing stress, getting enough sleep, staying active, and boosting your adrenal glands. Finally, we end with a series of delicious recipes that you can enjoy while achieving your weight-loss goals.

KEEPING WEIGHT OFF IN THE REAL WORLD

F ad diets come and go. Unfortunately, so do those unwanted pounds. Fortunately for you, this plan offers a safe and effective alternative to yo-yo dieting. As you follow the three-step plan and move from *belly fat* to *belly flat,* you will discover a lifetime approach to keeping your hormones balanced and your waistline trim. To keep you on track, here are some helpful hints and reminders:

- Keep your bio-identical progesterone cream and your supplements by your toothbrush so that incorporating them into your daily regimen quickly becomes automatic.
- Make a grocery list before you shop, and always shop on a full stomach. If you shop when you're hungry, you're more likely to be tempted by high-fat or high-calorie foods.
- Eat three meals a day and *never* skip breakfast. If you don't eat breakfast, your metabolism is more likely to

slow down to compensate for not receiving any new calories. In addition, you'll be more likely to experience low energy and food cravings later in the day.

- Eat slowly. It takes twenty minutes for your stomach to signal your brain that it is full. Try putting your fork down between bites, and take a drink of water to help you slow down.

- Do not eat in front of the television; when your attention is elsewhere, you're more likely to overeat.

- Avoid fast food, but when you have no other choice, order a grilled chicken "sandwich" without the bun or mayonnaise. Most fast-food chains now also offer some type of side salad or fruit cup. Don't eat the dressing. Sprinkle with lemon juice instead.

- When eating out, avoid croutons and order low-fat salad dressing on the side; drizzle sparingly.

- Also when eating out, ask for a double order of broccoli or asparagus and dress with lemon juice to substitute for a buttery potato or rice dish.

- Keep a large bowl of broccoli and cauliflower florets ready for cooking or snacking.

- Although the sample daily menus include only one afternoon snack, if you get hungry between breakfast and lunch, eat another recommended snack.

- Try to eat dinner before 7 PM, and then do not eat again until breakfast. Drink water with lemon until bedtime.

- Keep small sandwich bags of chopped carrots and celery and nuts in the refrigerator. Grab them for a quick snack when you are on the run.

- Keep a weekly weight-loss journal and diet diary (see Appendix A). Record your weight, symptoms of hormone imbalance, stress level, and exercise patterns. Measure your waistline circumference once a month.

Remember that the choices you make every minute of every day either work for you or against you. Unfortunately, people unknowingly sabotage their weight-loss efforts. There are four hidden saboteurs that can impact your weight: stress, lack of sleep, physical inactivity, and insufficient supplementation.

stress and your hormones

Although too much estrogen is the primary culprit that causes you to pack on those pounds, stress impacts the production of five other hormones that can influence your metabolism, your appetite, and your food cravings. Three of the five hormones are produced by the walnut-size adrenal glands located on top of each kidney. They are adrenaline, cortisol, and dehydroepiandrosterone (DHEA). The other two hormones are ghrelin and leptin, which are produced by a small area in the middle of the brain called the hypothalamus. If stress has disrupted the balance of one or more of these five hormones, you will tend to always be hungry and will never feel full no matter how much you eat. The result is more fat stored around your middle.

According to Tene T. Lewis, a health psychologist and lead researcher at Rush University Medical Center in Chicago, the pressures of a busy life can stimulate some bodies to conserve more fat. Dr. Lewis's team of researchers found that the more stressors that were reported, the more weight that was gained over four years. This weight gain was not attributable to other variables like diet or exercise.

What are life stressors? The list of stressors typically cited by patients include the following: daily time-management issues, juggling work and family, being laid off or fired, experiencing major money worries, losing a parent, going through a divorce, and dealing with difficult infants, angry teenagers, or aging parents. Can you identify?

How does stress impact hormone levels? When the brain perceives some form of danger, it signals the adrenal glands to pump out more adrenaline, often referred to as the "fight-or-flight" hormone. The sudden surge in adrenaline levels signals fat cells to quickly release energy. This energy rush stimulates flight. Once the body is out of danger, the brain continues to signal the adrenal glands that there is a temporary need to keep the adrenaline level elevated. Higher than normal adrenaline levels cause an increase in appetite, which encourages the body to eat more calories and replenish fat stores. In acute (short-term) stress situations, the adrenaline level will soon return to normal once the immediate appetite has been satisfied.

This brain-body hormone-stimulating phenomenon served human beings very well in times when people needed to avoid immediate dangers like being eaten by wolves or killed by invading armies. Today, however, the modern person in the United States is not frequently subjected to such immediate dangers.

Contemporary stressors, like worrying about paying the

mortgage, doing the jobs of three people, dealing with an unhappy marriage, or grappling with ongoing parenting issues, tend to be more long-term. A life stressor can be considered chronic if it persists for three or more months. Instead of pumping out more adrenaline, the adrenal glands respond to chronic stress by secreting more cortisol. Because chronic stress is ongoing, high cortisol levels do not subside until the stress is removed or the adrenal glands exhausted.

Over time, elevated cortisol levels can wreak havoc on your body. Sustained high cortisol levels destroy healthy muscle and bone, slow down healing and normal cell regeneration, deplete the necessary biochemicals to make other vital hormones, impair digestion, dull mental processes, interfere with healthy endocrine function, and weaken the immune system. If you are stressed out, high cortisol levels will also compromise your metabolism and cement more pounds around your middle.

In addition, when the adrenals are chronically overworked and are straining to maintain high cortisol levels, they lose the capacity to produce DHEA in sufficient amounts. DHEA is necessary to moderate the balance of hormones in your body. When DHEA is produced at optimal levels, it functions to promote the loss of body fat. Double-blind clinical trials have found 100 mg per day of DHEA to be effective in decreasing body fat in older men. Conversely, when the body's DHEA levels are insufficient, body fat is more difficult to budge.

Recently, a female patient named Shirley complained that she had gained fifteen pounds in the last nine months. She said she wouldn't be unhappy if she could only spread some of those pounds around to her "stick-skinny legs" or to her arms or chest. The problem was that all fifteen pounds had attached themselves to her middle.

Shirley reported that in the last eighteen months she had purchased a new home, moved across town and away from her familiar church and schools, and experienced the unanticipated death of a close childhood friend. There was no doubt that a combination of estrogen dominance, elevated cortisol levels, and insufficient DHEA levels were all contributing to why Shirley was packing those pounds around her middle.

I explained to Shirley that estrogen dominance can cause weight gain and bloating, and that deep abdominal tissue has up to four times the number of cortisol receptors than any other area of the body. When the body is under stress, the cells in the abdomen are the most aggressive in responding to increased cortisol levels. The result is a biochemically driven accumulation of extra abdominal flab.

Six months after her first consultation, Shirley returned and said the following:

When I first came to you complaining that my gut had become a fat magnet, you recommended that I start a regimen that would include bio-identical progesterone cream, foods and supplements to support hormone balance, and a practice of consciously relaxing three times a day. I bought into your approach to eliminating my condition of estrogen dominance, but I thought the whole idea of de-stressing to support hormone balance was hokey, so I just blew that part off.

In two months I lost eight pounds and was excited. Then for the next two months, no more weight loss. I was discouraged, but I remembered what you had said about how stress can sabotage hormone balance, so I decided to give relaxation a try. I began to practice conscious breathing every time I came to a red light. Also, I set aside ten minutes every morning to just sit quietly and imagine myself at the beach. In four weeks, those last seven pounds I wanted to lose just melted away.

how stressed are you?

The list shown in Table 6-1 is adapted from the work of mental health experts Thomas H. Holmes and Richard H. Rahe. It's very useful for obtaining a snapshot of your overall stress level.

Note that each stress-inducing event has been assigned a life-change unit (LCU). To quantify your stress level, first circle all the life events that you have experienced within the last twelve months. Next, add up the corresponding LCUs. Once you have your LCU total, find your stress-level category. Finally, read how your stress level is linked with hormone imbalance.

from belly fat to belly flat

Table 6-1. Stress-Inducing Events

Life Event	LCU	Life Event	LCU
Death of spouse	100	Children leaving home	29
Divorce	73	Trouble with difficult teenagers	29
Marital separation	65	Outstanding personal achievement	28
Jail term	63	Spouse begins or stops work	26
Death of a close family member	63	Starting or ending school	26
Personal injury or illness	53	Change in living conditions	25
Marriage	50	Revision of personal habits	24
Being fired from work	47	(dress, manners, associations)	
Reconciliation with spouse	45	Trouble with boss	23
Retirement	45	Change in work hours	20
Change in health of a family member	44	or conditions	
Illness or change in care needs of a parent	40	Change in residence	20
		Change in school	20
Sexual difficulties	39	Change in recreational activities	19
Addition of a family member	39	Change in religious activities	19
Major business readjustment	39	Change in social activities	18
Major change in financial state	38	Mortgage or loan under $15,000	17
Death of a close friend	37	Change in sleeping habits	16
Changing to a different line of work	36	Change in number of family	15
Change in frequency of arguments with spouse	35	gatherings	
		Change in eating habits	15
New loan for major purchase over $15,000	31	Vacation	13
		Christmas	12
Foreclosure on a mortgage or loan	30	Minor violation of the law	11
Major change in responsibilities at work	29		
		LCU Total Score: _____	

Here is what your LCU total score reveals:

- If your total is 0–150: At the moment, your stress level is low. The chance of your stress triggering a hormone imbalance is also low. Good for you.
- If your total is 150–300: You have borderline high stress. Your risk for a stress-related hormone imbalance is moderate.
- If your total is more than 300: Warning! You have a high stress level. Your chance of having a stress-related hormone imbalance is significant.

Because the average person's life is full of responsibilities and complications, it is just not reasonable to think that you can completely eliminate stress as a factor. There are, however, tools and strategies that can help you to better cope with day-to-day stress. Proactive stress management has been shown to decrease the body's susceptibility to the fight-or-flight surge of adrenal hormones.

hormone-healthy habit: beat stress

Although de-stressing is part of the prescription for restoring and maintaining hormone balance, setting aside time for yourself will be one of your greatest challenges. Experiment with different approaches to determine which ones will work best for you.

breathe

A common response to our hurried and fragmented lives is physical tension in the body and shallow breathing through the chest. Simply making a conscious effort to breathe more deeply and slowly can elicit a relaxation response to counteract your automatic stress response.

Try to set aside five minutes three times a day to close your door, turn off the phone, and just focus on inhalation and exhalation. Some people accomplish this best when they are naturally sequestered; for instance, in a car or on the toilet. Try the following technique:

- Put your hand under your belly button and focus on moving your breath down through your belly rather than up through your chest.
- Breathe in through your nose for a count of four.
- Hold for a count of three.
- Exhale through your mouth for a count of four.

Take any routine interruption that you find annoying in life and "reprogram" it as a cue to pause and breathe more consciously. Red lights, e-mail message alerts, and being put on hold during a telephone call can all serve this function.

meditate

For most of us, our minds are busy even when our bodies are still. When you use meditation to elicit the relaxation response, you turn your attention inward, concentrating on a repetitive positive thought, prayer, or image to reduce the reactivity of your thoughts.

Some patients have told me that they meditate by repeating a mantra of love or peace with each exhalation; others say that they recite a memorized prayer; or personally, I picture myself on the shores of a beach listening to the ebb and flow of the waves. I encourage you to develop your own personal meditation to help your body and mind begin to quiet down so that a state of physiological and mental rest can ensue.

Begin by setting aside ten minutes each day to meditate. Do your best to find a quiet space where you won't be disturbed. You can meditate in any position, but the best way is to sit up with a straight back or in a comfortable chair. To help you fully relax and eliminate the need to look at your watch, set a timer or gentle alarm.

visualize

A psychologist I know well has a fun technique to reduce your reaction to stressful people. He suggests that whenever you are around someone who is causing you to tense up or feel anxious, you should visualize that person's face on a tiny mouse's body with really big ears. Then, he suggests, imagine yourself taking a big broom to firmly and efficiently swish that mouse away.

Another visualization technique is to imagine that your stress has a shape and form and has attached itself like gum to the bottom of your shoe. Visualize yourself taking off your shoe, peeling off that nasty stress, and throwing it in the garbage. The goal is to create an image of stress as something you can get rid of.

Finally, simply close your eyes and take yourself on a trip to the most peaceful place you have ever been or read about. Imagine how the air feels against your skin and how restful your mind is while you are there. When you reenter your true surroundings, you will most likely feel refreshed from your brief mental vacation.

sleep disturbances and your hormones

Stress can cause you to toss and turn at night. Stress-induced insomnia can impact two hormones that function to stimulate and control your appetite: ghrelin, the hormone that pumps through your body when you feel hungry, and leptin, the hormone that tells you that you are full and to stop eating.

In the long-term Wisconsin Sleep Cohort Study, men and women who routinely slept eight hours nightly were compared to those who slept five hours or less. The findings indicated that those sleeping five hours or less had a 15 percent higher level of ghrelin, the hormone signaling hunger, and a 16 percent lower level of leptin, the hormone signally fullness.

According to Peter Kilpton, health journalist and author of *Less Sleep Can Equal More Weight*, when you are deprived of sleep, the production of ghrelin and leptin are affected, and not in a positive way. Researchers have concluded that a sleep deficit leads to elevated levels of ghrelin in your system. If you are not getting enough sleep, your body responds by telling you that you are hungrier. Furthermore, when you do eat, it will take you longer to feel full and satisfied. This is because the amount of leptin in your system has decreased. The combination of elevated ghrelin (making you feel constantly hungry) and decreased leptin (telling you that you still aren't full) will wreak havoc on your waistline.

hormone-healthy habit: snooze and lose

Substantial medical evidence suggests that there is a strong link between sleep and weight. Researchers say that how much you sleep, and quite possibly the quality of your sleep, can silently orchestrate a symphony of hormonal activity that is tied to your appetite.

According to Michael Breus, a faculty member of the Atlanta School of Sleep Medicine and director of the Sleep Disorders Centers of Southeastern Lung Care in Atlanta, a lack of sleep drives leptin levels down, which means that you don't feel as satisfied after you eat. It also causes ghrelin levels to rise, which means that your appetite is stimulated, so you want more food.

Because estrogen dominance frequently causes insomnia or fitful sleeping as a result of hot flashes and night sweats, using bio-identical progesterone cream and eating foods to reduce your estrogen load should help to promote a healthy sleeping pattern. However, you still have to make the choice to stop whatever you are doing and get into bed early enough to allow yourself eight hours of sleep.

physical inactivity and your hormones

Numerous studies in the last several decades have confirmed that physical activity has a positive effect on longevity and mortality and that a lack of physical activity is associated with an increased risk of disease and disability. Regular physical activity helps to regulate cortisol production, making it less likely that surging cortisol levels will contribute to both a constant feeling of anxiety and an ever-expanding waistline.

hormone-healthy habit: find a way to move

In order to commit yourself to a regular fitness program, you must set goals that you know you can meet. If you do not currently exercise, start by planning to simply move your body thirty to forty minutes each day. Do something you enjoy: walk, dance, ride a bike, swim, do yoga, attend an aerobics class, or jump rope. This might sound harsh, but *if you are too busy to exercise every day, then every day you are busy dying.*

boosting your adrenal glands

The adrenal glands are the main site of stress damage in the body. Certain supplements can nourish depleted adrenal glands while encouraging adrenal cortex secretions, which help to maintain optimal hormone balance.

In addition to the supplements described in Chapter 5, I designed an Adrenal Boost formula to increase overall energy and decrease fatigue. It is helpful for people who are under stress because it supports the glands that are responsible for energy flow. Anyone whose adrenal system is depressed by stress should also take 7-keto DHEA.

The ingredients in the Adrenal Boost formula are vitamin C, vitamin B_6, pantothenic acid, deglycerized licorice root, Mexican wild yam root, schizandra berry, *Eleutherococcus senticosus* root, stinging nettle leaf, trimethylglycine, special plant cellulose, natural silica, vegetable stearate, and magnesium stearate. I recommend that people dealing with chronic (long-term) stress take one capsule every morning and every night if they need it.

You should not take Adrenal Boost, however, if you have high blood pressure, because licorice root can elevate blood pressure.

In summary, you do not have to allow stress and/or poor lifestyle choices to upset your hormone balance. A proactive regimen of self-care is the best way to vaporize those weight-loss saboteurs that lurk in the corners of your everyday life. Even though most of us can't take a week a month just to chill out and can't afford a full-time housekeeper, chauffeur, or chef, we can make simple (and free) adjustments in our everyday lives to manage daily stress, enjoy a good night's sleep, get some exercise, and supplement a fatigued adrenal system.

Hormone balance is a process, not a fixed state. What works to balance your hormones in your thirties and early forties might not work as you approach your late forties and early fifties. The production of your hormones will continue to shift and decline with age.

About 80 percent of women and men will never need anything more than over-the-counter bio-identical progesterone, our recommended regimen of foods and supplements, and a practice of hormone-healthy life habits to maintain optimal hormone balance. However, with age, approximately 20 percent of women and men will suffer a decline in estrogen and/or testosterone production that will require treatment. They will need the help of a knowledgeable physician and a compounding pharmacist. For those who are on a comprehensive bio-identical hormone replacement regimen, it will be critical that they stick to their diet and take their supplements if they want to lose their belly fat and keep it off for good.

THE 80-20 RULE

In this chapter I introduce you to what I call the 80-20 rule of bio-identical hormone replacement therapy (BHRT) and long-term weight management. Approximately 80 percent of men and women find that over-the-counter bio-identical progesterone cream, combined with foods and supplements to support hormone balance, is all they need to get and keep those unwanted pounds off. However, the other 20 percent discover that the pounds begin to creep back on and realize that they need a bit more help.

How will you know if you are one of the 20 percent who needs extra bio-identical hormone support? Your body will tell you. Typically, this will happen in your late forties and fifties.

Pam had been my patient for twelve years. When she first came in at age thirty-nine, she was twenty-five pounds over-weight and experiencing constant headaches, fatigue, and bloating. After following the three-step plan for just a month, her symptoms went away. She lost all the excess weight in four months and, by continuing on the plan, kept those pounds off. Then, when she was fifty-one years old, Pam was back in the office for her annual exam, and she wasn't happy.

"What has happened to your bio-identical progesterone cream?" she asked. "I am still eating all the foods to reduce my estrogen load and taking my supplements, but I have gained nineteen pounds in nine months. It's got to be a change in your cream!"

Pam complained that she was having night sweats and hot flashes. She also reported that she had not had a period for eleven months. When a woman has not had a period for twelve months, she is officially menopausal. Pam was on that cusp, and the production of her other sex hormones had declined to a point that additional help might be necessary. The progesterone cream had not changed, but the balance among her other hormones had.

one size does not fit all

As stated in the previous chapter, hormone balance is a process, not a fixed state. Although progesterone production is the first to decline in women, with age the production of estrogen and testosterone will also decline. This means that the hormone replacement that works for you today might not work for you five years from now.

How will you know if you are one of the 20 percent who also needs to address a shift in estrogen and testosterone production? Your symptoms will be your first clue. If symptoms of hormone imbalance persist or return when you are using a regimen of bio-identical progesterone cream and foods and supplements to support hormone balance, then the balance of your other hormones has also shifted and will require attention.

Women in their thirties or forties who enter abrupt artificial menopause as a result of a complete hysterectomy should be placed on a full regimen of bio-identical hormone replacement. As they age, some women sail through natural menopause with the help of the three-step plan only. Other women have a flare-up of symptoms that require additional hormone supplementation. As for men, if they experience a progressive decline in libido in their late forties and early fifties, they should work with a physician to determine if they are candidates for bio-identical testosterone replacement.

when you will need a doctor

A doctor will have to order either a saliva or a blood serum test to analyze all your hormone levels. Once a doctor has determined which hormones are deficient, he or she can write a prescription for a formulation of BHRT to address your unique needs.

Patients come to see me from all over the world because it's not always easy to find a physician who has experience diagnosing hormone imbalances and BHRT as the preferred treatment. BHRT is not yet taught in medical schools, and most physicians remain uneducated about it.

However, since the World Health Institute has begun detailing the significant health risks of synthetic hormone replacement, this trend is shifting. In the last several years, hundreds of doctors have attended national continuing medical education forums on the subject of BHRT. In most cases, these doctors have been prodded by their patients' demands for safe and effective alternatives; as a result, these doctors have taken the initiative to educate themselves.

If you do not know a physician in your area who is proficient in BHRT, ask your local compounding pharmacist (see below). Appendix C also offers resources for locating a physician.

why you will need a compounding pharmacy

Once your doctor determines exactly which hormones are deficient, your prescription will have to be filled in a compounding pharmacy. Although some pharmaceutical companies are now manufacturing standard dosages of BHRT, it is more typical for a doctor to write a prescription for the exact amount of the hormones that your body needs. A compounding pharmacist will then mix your individualized prescription on site.

If you have never had your prescriptions filled by a compounding pharmacist, here are some facts you should know:

• Every compounding pharmacy is licensed and inspected by the State Pharmacy Board.

• Compounding pharmacists are educated and trained to provide information about the formulation of bioidentical hormones. In many cases, they help to educate the physician on dosing and delivery options.

- All materials used in compounding formulations are subject to FDA inspection and the agency's Good Manufacturing Procedures code.

- The International Academy of Compounding Pharmacists (IACP) and the Professional Compounding Centers for America (PCCA) are two excellent resources to help you or your physician locate a compounding pharmacy in your area. Their contact information is provided in Appendix C.

If you are one of the 20 percent who require a more comprehensive plan of BHRT, you will still need help to win your battle of the bulge. Also remember: You should never take any form of estrogen therapy, even if it is bio-identical, without also taking bio-identical progesterone.

If you are on any form of bio-identical estrogen replacement, it might seem counterproductive to continue to eat foods and take supplements to reduce your estrogen load. However, it is not. In fact, by continuing to eat foods that reduce your estrogen load and take supplements that support overall hormone balance, you can positively influence how the estrogen is metabolized in your body.

The names for the three most commonly prescribed formulations of bio-identical estrogen are tri-est, bi-est, and estradiol. Tri-est is a combination of the three estrogens you learned about earlier: estrone (E1), estradiol (E2), and estriol (E3). Bi-est is a combination of E2 and E3, and estradiol is simple E2. Just like the estrogen produced by your ovaries, bio-identical estrogen returns to the liver to be metabolized after it completes its required activity within the body. There it is broken down into different enzymatic pathways. The first, the 2-hydroxy pathway, results in "good" estrogen metabolites. The second, the 16-hydroxy pathway, produces one of the "bad" estrogen metabolites, which results in an increased risk of cancer. The third, the 4-hydroxy pathway, is associated with an even higher rate of cancer.

It seems obvious that you should want more "good" estrogens than "bad" estrogens. Foods and supplements can influence which enzymatic pathway estrogen goes down. For instance, you have learned that cruciferous vegetables act as a catalyst to pull estrogen down a benign pathway to 2-hydroxyestrone, thus decreasing the levels of the carcinogenic 4- and 16-alpha hydroxyestrones, the "bad" estrogens. In addition, the supplement DIM supports the activity of enzymes that improve estrogen metabolism by increasing the levels of 2-hydroxyestrone, the "good" estrogen.

If you are on a more comprehensive BHRT regimen that includes bio-identical estrogen, it is essential that you stick to this plan. When you do, you will continue to reduce your unhealthy estrogen load, support overall hormone balance, protect yourself from hormone-dependent cancers, and keep your belly flat for life.

THE "FLAT BELLY FOR LIFE" RECIPE COLLECTION

MAIN DISHES. 122

VEGETABLE DISHES 151

SALADS, SALAD DRESSINGS,
AND SNACKS 171

MAIN DISHES

Asparagus Omelet

4 egg whites
¼ teaspoon salt
4 egg yolks
Dash of pepper
1 cup 1% milk fat cottage cheese
1½ tablespoons extra-virgin olive oil
6 asparagus spears, trimmed and slightly
    steamed

    Preheat oven to 350°F. Beat egg whites until frothy. Add salt and beat until stiff. Beat yolks until thick and lemon colored; add pepper and cottage cheese and beat until well blended. Fold egg whites into yolks. Heat olive oil in a 10-inch iron skillet; pour in omelet and cook approximately 3 minutes, until the bottom is lightly browned. Top with asparagus spears and finish cooking in the oven for 15 minutes or until a knife inserted in the center comes out clean. Makes 2 servings.

NUTRITION FACTS

Amount Per Serving: Calories 340 – Calories from Fat 190 – Total Fat 21 g
Saturated Fat 6 g – Cholesterol 420 mg – Sodium 840 mg – Total Carbohydrate 11 g
Dietary Fiber 2 g – Sugars 7 g – Protein 26 g – Calcium 25% DV

Baked Fish with Basil

Organic nonstick cooking spray
6 (6-ounce) fish filets
1 cup chopped fresh basil
¼ cup extra-virgin olive oil
2 tablespoons minced garlic
1 tablespoon lemon juice
Salt and pepper to taste
1 lemon, sliced

Preheat oven to 350°F. Place fish filets in baking dish that you've sprayed with organic nonstick cooking spray. Combine basil, olive oil, garlic, and lemon juice in small bowl. Mix well and spoon evenly over fish. Add salt and pepper. Bake for 20–25 minutes, until the fish flakes easily with a fork. Garnish with lemon slices and serve. Makes 6 servings.

NUTRITION FACTS

Amount Per Serving: Calories 250 – Calories from Fat 110 – Total Fat 12 g
Saturated Fat 2.5 g – Cholesterol 85 mg – Sodium 90 mg – Total Carbohydrate 1 g
Dietary Fiber 0 g – Sugars 0 g – Protein 35 g – Calcium 4% DV

Black Beanofritos

2 cups (one 16-ounce can) black beans
1 medium tomato, chopped
1 small onion, minced
Salt and pepper to taste
1 avocado
⅓ cup plain low-fat yogurt
4 low-fat whole-wheat tortilla wraps
2 tablespoons chopped fresh cilantro
Dash of Tabasco (optional)

In a medium skillet, sauté the black beans with the tomato and onion until the vegetables are soft and the beans are hot. Add salt and pepper while mixture is cooking. Peel the avocado, mash with a potato masher, and mix well with yogurt. Remove bean mixture from skillet and drain any liquid. Using the potato masher, mash the bean mixture and then spoon it evenly onto the center of each tortilla, placed on a plate or platter. Fold the tortilla over, top with with a tablespoon of the avocado-yogurt mixture, and sprinkle with fresh cilantro (and a dash of Tabasco if desired) before serving. Makes 4 servings.

NUTRITION FACTS

Amount Per Serving: Calories 340 – Calories from Fat 90 – Total Fat 9 g – Saturated Fat 1 g – Cholesterol 0 mg – Sodium 190 mg – Total Carbohydrate 51 g Dietary Fiber 11 g – Sugars 4 g – Protein 14 g – Calcium 6% DV

Cauliflower and Turkey Bacon Soup

2½ cups chopped white onion
3 tablespoons extra-virgin olive oil
2 teaspoons ground cumin
1½ teaspoons ground fennel
2 cups minute brown rice
4 cups hot water
5 cups chopped cauliflower
1 cup grated carrots
1 tablespoon vegetable bouillon powder or
   1 bouillon cube
2 tablespoons fresh lemon juice
Salt and pepper to taste
5 slices cooked turkey bacon, crumbled

In a large soup pot on medium heat, sauté the onion in the olive oil for 5–10 minutes until translucent. Stir in the cumin, fennel, and brown rice. Add hot water. Cover and bring to a boil. Add the cauliflower, carrots, and bouillon, and return to a boil before lowering the heat to simmer for 10–15 minutes. Remove from heat.

In a blender, puree the vegetables and broth until smooth. Add the lemon juice and salt and pepper. Return to soup pan and reheat. Top with crumbled turkey bacon just before serving. Makes 6–8 servings.

NUTRITION FACTS

Amount Per Serving: Calories 310 – Calories from Fat 100 – Total Fat 11 g
Saturated Fat 2 g – Cholesterol 10 mg – Sodium 420 mg – Total Carbohydrate 44 g
Dietary Fiber 7 g – Sugars 7 g – Protein 9 g – Calcium 6% DV

Cauliflower Crab Cakes

2 cups crabmeat
2 cups cooked and mashed cauliflower
⅓ cup minced celery
⅓ cup minced onion
1 tablespoon parsley
2 eggs, beaten
Extra-virgin olive oil or grapeseed oil (for
    sautéing)

Combine all ingredients in a large bowl, except the olive oil. Form into 6 patties and chill in refrigerator for at least 1 hour. Brown in skillet lightly coated with olive oil. Makes 6 servings.

NUTRITION FACTS

Amount Per Serving: Calories 160 – Calories from Fat 40 – Total Fat 4.5 g – Saturated Fat 1 g – Cholesterol 140 mg – Sodium 500 mg – Total Carbohydrate 6 g Dietary Fiber 2 g – Sugars 2 g – Protein 24 g – Calcium 10% DV

Chicken and Asparagus
Lettuce Wraps

1 cup asparagus, washed and trimmed
4 (6-ounce) skinless, boneless chicken breast
halves
2 tablespoons extra-virgin olive oil
1 tablespoon rice vinegar
1 tablespoon low-sodium soy sauce
1 teaspoon grated fresh ginger
½ teaspoon grated orange rind
2 teaspoons minced garlic
½ cup grated carrots
1 head romaine lettuce

Chop the asparagus into pieces that are, at most, ⅛ inch
long. Slice the chicken breast into thin strips. Mix the olive
oil, vinegar, soy sauce, ginger, orange rind, and garlic in
a bowl. Add the chicken and asparagus and chill for 1
hour. Pour into a skillet, add carrots, and brown for 10–12
minutes, until the chicken is done. Drop a large spoonful of
the cooked mixture onto the center of each lettuce leaf. Roll
like a burrito and serve. Makes 6 servings.

NUTRITION FACTS

Amount Per Serving: Calories 250 – Calories from Fat 80 – Total Fat 9 g – Saturated
Fat 2 g – Cholesterol 95 mg – Sodium 190 mg – Total Carbohydrate 4 g
Dietary Fiber 1 g – Sugars 2 g – Protein 36 g – Calcium 4% DV

Colorful Turkey Casserole

1 (3-pound) turkey breast
1 teaspoon salt
½ teaspoon pepper
½ teaspoon oregano
½ teaspoon rosemary
Extra-virgin olive oil
2 cups raw grated carrots
2 cups raw chopped asparagus
1 yellow pepper, sliced
1 16-ounce can tomato sauce
2 cloves garlic
2 cups steamed spinach

Preheat oven to 325°F. Cut turkey into strips. Sprinkle with salt, pepper, oregano, and rosemary, then brown in a skillet in olive oil. Place the pieces in a casserole dish that is very lightly greased with olive oil. Sauté carrots, asparagus, and yellow pepper in skillet until soft. Remove from heat and stir in tomato sauce, garlic, and spinach. Pour over chicken and toss. Bake uncovered for 1 hour. Makes 6 servings.

NUTRITION FACTS

Amount Per Serving: Calories 440 – Calories from Fat 20 – Total Fat 2.5 g
Saturated Fat 0.5 g – Cholesterol 190 mg – Sodium 980 mg – Total Carbohydrate 28 g
Dietary Fiber 6 g – Sugars 7 g – Protein 75 g – Calcium 25% DV

Favorite Feta Frittata

1 pound spinach leaves, washed and chopped
9 large eggs
2 tablespoons skim milk
⅓ cup grated Parmesan cheese
2 tablespoons chopped sun-dried tomatoes
Salt and freshly ground pepper to taste
1 medium onion, chopped (about 1 cup)
1 tablespoon extra-virgin olive oil
1 large clove garlic, minced
3 ounces reduced-fat feta cheese

Preheat oven to 400°F. Cook spinach in ¼ cup water in covered saucepan until just wilted (a couple minutes). Drain water and set aside. In a mixing bowl, whisk together eggs, milk, and Parmesan cheese. Add tomatoes and sprinkle with salt and pepper. Set aside.

Sauté onion in olive oil in an oven-safe skillet until translucent, about 2 minutes on medium-high heat. Add garlic and sauté a minute more. Add cooked spinach and mix with onion and garlic. Spread spinach mixture evenly on the bottom of the skillet. Pour the egg mixture over the spinach mixture. Use a spatula to lift up the spinach mixture along the sides of the pan to let the egg mixture flow underneath. Sprinkle bits of feta cheese over the top of the frittata mixture.

When the mixture is about half set, put the whole pan in the oven. Bake 13–15 minutes, until frittata is puffy and golden. Remove from oven and let cool for several minutes. Makes 5 servings.

NUTRITION FACTS

Amount Per Serving: Calories 250 – Calories from Fat 150 – Total Fat 16 g
Saturated Fat 6 g – Cholesterol 390 mg – Sodium 540 mg – Total Carbohydrate 7 g
Dietary Fiber 3 g – Sugars 3 g – Protein 20 g – Calcium 25% DV

Fish New Orleans Style

3 bay leaves
3 sprigs fresh thyme or 1 tablespoon dried thyme
1 clove garlic
½ teaspoon salt
½ teaspoon pepper
A pinch of cayenne pepper
3 pounds white fish, such as flounder
   or grouper
1 cup chopped broccoli
1 cup chopped tomatoes
½ cup chopped green onions (scallions)
Extra-virgin olive oil
1 lemon

Preheat oven to 350°F. Chop bay leaves, thyme, and garlic very fine. Add salt, pepper, and cayenne. Rub the fish inside and out with this mixture and place in a baking dish. Sauté the broccoli, tomatoes, and scallions in olive oil. Pour over fish and bake for 30 minutes. Squeeze lemon onto fish before serving. Makes 6 servings.

NUTRITION FACTS

Amount Per Serving: Calories 220 – Calories from Fat 25 – Total Fat 3 g – Saturated Fat 0.5 g – Cholesterol 110 mg – Sodium 390 mg – Total Carbohydrate 4 g Dietary Fiber 1 g – Sugars 1 g – Protein 43 g – Calcium 6% DV

Garlic Chickpeas and Pasta

1 (16-ounce) can chickpeas (garbanzo beans)
1 (8-ounce) can crushed tomatoes with basil
1 cup steamed broccoli, chopped
3 tablespoons chopped garlic
1 cup water
½ teaspoon extra-virgin olive oil
Salt and pepper to taste
1 cup uncooked whole-grain pasta

In large bowl, mix chickpeas, tomatoes, broccoli, and garlic. Add water, olive oil, salt, and pepper to a large pot and bring to a boil. Add pasta and cook according to the time recommended on the package. Remove pasta, drain, and toss with chickpea mixture. Serve immediately. Makes 6 servings.

NUTRITION FACTS

Amount Per Serving: Calories 210 – Calories from Fat 25 – Total Fat 2.5 g – Saturated Fat 0 g – Cholesterol 0 mg – Sodium 135 mg – Total Carbohydrate 39 g Dietary Fiber 9 g – Sugars 6 g – Protein 11 g – Calcium 6% DV

Grilled Fish with Citrus Marinade

¼ cup extra-virgin olive oil
2 tablespoons grapefruit juice
3 tablespoons lime juice
Salt and pepper to taste
4 (6-ounce) fish filets

Combine olive oil, grapefruit juice, lime juice, salt, and pepper. Pour over fish and marinate in refrigerateor for 2 or more hours. Grill and serve. Makes 4 servings.

NUTRITION FACTS

Amount Per Serving: Calories 200 – Calories from Fat 60 – Total Fat 6 g – Saturated Fat 1.5 g – Cholesterol 85 mg – Sodium 90 mg – Total Carbohydrate 0 g Dietary Fiber 0 g – Sugars 0 g – Protein 34 g – Calcium 2% DV

Grilled Salmon with Dill and Lemon

2 tablespoons dill
1 teaspoon garlic powder
4 tablespoons extra-virgin olive oil
2 tablespoons white wine vinegar
    with tarragon
Juice of 2 lemons
4 (1-inch thick) salmon steaks, 4 ounces each

Mix dill, garlic powder, olive oil, vinegar, and lemon juice. Pour mixture over salmon steaks and marinate in the refrigerator for at least 2 hours, turning at least once. Place salmon on hot grill and cook 3–5 minutes on each side. Makes 4 servings.

NUTRITION FACTS

Amount Per Serving: Calories 280 – Calories from Fat 130 – Total Fat 14 g
Saturated Fat 2 g – Cholesterol 95 mg – Sodium 75 mg – Total Carbohydrate 1 g
Dietary Fiber 0 g – Sugars 0 g – Protein 34 g – Calcium 2% DV

Lemon Hot Fish

Organic nonstick cooking spray
6 (4-ounce) filets of white fish
5 cloves garlic, chopped
1 cup fresh spinach
1 cup cauliflower, sliced thin
2–3 bay leaves
1 cup lemon juice
½ cup rice wine vinegar
2 tablespoons Tabasco
2 tablespoons extra-virgin olive oil
Salt and pepper to taste
2 tablespoons toasted flaxseed
1 lemon cut into wedges
Fresh parsley

Preheat oven to 350°F. Place fish in a baking pan that you've sprayed with organic nonstick cooking spray. Cover with garlic, spinach, cauliflower, and bay leaves. In a small bowl, mix the lemon juice, vinegar, Tabasco, olive oil, salt, and pepper. Pour over fish. Bake covered for 30 minutes, stirring vegetables twice so they absorb the juice evenly. Then bake uncovered for another 15 minutes. Remove and place on serving platter. Remove bay leaves. Sprinkle with toasted flaxseed and garnish with lemons and parsley. Makes 6 servings.

NUTRITION FACTS

Amount Per Serving: Calories 160 – Calories from Fat 45 – Total Fat 5 g – Saturated Fat 1 g – Cholesterol 55 mg – Sodium 75 mg – Total Carbohydrate 4 g Dietary Fiber 2 g – Sugars 1 g – Protein 24 g – Calcium 4% DV

Lentil, Carrot, and Turnip Stew

1 cup red lentils
4 large carrots, sliced
1–2 large onions, chopped
1 tablespoon minced garlic
Extra-virgin olive oil
1 large (16-ounce) can tomatoes or 8–10 fresh
     ones, chopped
1 (16-ounce) bag frozen chopped turnips
2–3 sprigs parsley or 1 teaspoon dried parsley
Salt, pepper, and Tabasco to taste

Thoroughly rinse the red lentils in a strainer and remove any small black rocks that are sometimes found among them. Boil the lentils in a large pot for about 20 minutes, in enough water so that the lentils can expand to roughly four times their original size. Add carrots and boil for 5 more minutes. Brown the onion and garlic in olive oil in a skillet. Add onion mixture to the pot. Toss in the can of tomatoes (with the liquid) and add the turnips and parsley. Cook over low to medium heat for 15 minutes, stirring occasionally so the lentils don't stick to the bottom of the pan. Add salt, pepper, and Tabasco to taste. Serve in bowls. Makes 4 servings.

NUTRITION FACTS

Amount Per Serving: Calories 260 – Calories from Fat 15 – Total Fat 1.5 g – Saturated Fat 0 g – Cholesterol 0 mg – Sodium 115 mg – Total Carbohydrate 52 g Dietary Fiber 17 g – Sugars 20 g – Protein 15 g – Calcium 15% DV

Nest of Beans and Greens

1 cup dried lima beans
2 hard-boiled eggs, finely chopped
3 tablespoons extra-virgin olive oil
1 bunch of turnip, collard, or mustard greens
  (about 2 pounds) or 1 (16-ounce) package
  frozen greens
Juice of 1 lemon
Salt, pepper, vinegar, and crushed pepper flakes
  (optional) to taste

Soak and cook lima beans according to the directions on the package. Drain. Add the eggs to the beans and use a potato masher to mash into a paste. Use the olive oil sparingly if some moisture is needed. Set aside. Saute the greens in a medium saucepan until tender but still green. Make a nest of greens on each plate. Put 2 tablespoons of the lima bean mash in the center. Sprinkle lemon juice and season as desired with salt, pepper, vinegar, and red pepper flakes. Makes 4 servings.

NUTRITION FACTS

Amount Per Serving: Calories 310 – Calories from Fat 130 – Total Fat 14 g
Saturated Fat 2.5 g – Cholesterol 105 mg – Sodium 85 mg – Total Carbohydrate 35 g
Dietary Fiber 15 g – Sugars 1 g – Protein 16 g – Calcium 35% DV

Open-Faced Veggie Cheeseburger

¼ pound green beans
½ cup cracked wheat
1 small zucchini
1 small carrot, peeled
½ Granny Smith apple, peeled
½ cup canned chickpeas, rinsed and drained
1 tablespoon minced onion
1 tablespoon minced garlic
½ teaspoon curry powder
½ teaspoon chili powder
Salt and pepper to taste
2 tablespoons extra-virgin olive oil
½ cup grated Cheddar cheese
½ cup whole-grain bread crumbs
Sliced tomato, onion, and whole-grain
    hamburger buns (optional)

Cook green beans in boiling water until tender but crisp. Drain and chop very fine. Cook cracked wheat in 1 cup boiling water for 1 minute. Remove from heat and cover. Grate the zucchini, carrot, and apple; place on a paper towel and squeeze out excess moisture. Combine with the chopped beans.

In a food processor, blend the chickpeas, onions, garlic, curry powder, chili powder, salt, pepper, and olive oil until smooth. Add to the green bean mixture.

Drain the cracked wheat in a strainer, pressing with the back of a spoon to extract excess liquid. Add to the vegetables. Stir in the cheese and add the bread crumbs. Refrigerate for 1 hour.

Shape into four burgers. Cook 3 minutes on each side on a grill lightly brushed with olive oil. Serve as is or on ½ hamburger bun; top with tomato and onion if desired. Makes 4 servings.

NUTRITION FACTS

Amount Per Serving: Calories 290 – Calories from Fat 120 – Total Fat 13 g
Saturated Fat 4.5 g – Cholesterol 15 mg – Sodium 200 mg – Total Carbohydrate 33 g
Dietary Fiber 6 g – Sugars 5 g – Protein 10 g – Calcium 15% DV

Orange-Ginger Salmon

1 cup extra-virgin olive oil
½ cup orange juice
1 tablespoon minced garlic
4 1-inch (5-ounce) salmon steaks
Fresh ginger slivers

Mix the olive oil, orange juice, and garlic. Pour the mixture over the salmon and marinate at least 2 hours (or refrigerate overnight). Preheat the oven to broil. Broil the fish 2–3 inches from the heating element for 5 minutes, then turn and broil on the other side. You may also heat any saved marinade and spoon over the fish just before serving. Makes 4 servings.

NUTRITION FACTS

Amount Per Serving: Calories 310 – Calories from Fat 160 – Total Fat 18 g
Saturated Fat 2.5 g – Cholesterol 95 mg – Sodium 75 mg – Total Carbohydrate 2 g
Dietary Fiber 0 g – Sugars 1 g – Protein 34 g – Calcium 2% DV

Pan-Roasted Fish
with Parsley and Turkey Bacon

8 slices turkey bacon
3 tablespoons extra-virgin olive oil
1 cup baby portabella mushrooms, sliced
1 tablespoon minced garlic
2 tablespoons minced parsley
4 (6-ounce) fish filets (or 1½–2 pounds
   whole fish)
Salt and pepper to taste
Lemon wedges

Cut the turkey bacon into 1-inch pieces and sauté in skillet in 1 tablespoon olive oil for 2–3 minutes; add the mushrooms and cook about 5 more minutes. Stir in the garlic and parsley and remove from heat. Put the remaining 2 tablespoons of olive oil in a skillet and add the fish filets. Cook on low to medium heat for 10–15 minutes or until a fork or knife easily penetrates the flesh. Pour the bacon mixture over the fish and let simmer. Add salt and pepper. Serve immediately and garnish with lemon wedges. Makes 4 servings.

NUTRITION FACTS

Amount Per Serving: Calories 380 – Calories from Fat 190 – Total Fat 21 g
Saturated Fat 5 g – Cholesterol 115 mg – Sodium 740 mg – Total Carbohydrate 3 g
Dietary Fiber 1 g – Sugars 1 g – Protein 43 g – Calcium 2% DV

Quick Turkey-Stuffed Cabbage

1 pound ground turkey
1 large onion, chopped
1 cup brown rice, uncooked
¼ cup fresh mint, chopped, or
    1 tablespoon dried mint
1 egg, beaten
2 (14-ounce) cans chicken broth
Salt and pepper to taste
2 tablespoons extra-virgin olive oil
1 medium cabbage
2 tablespoons flaxseed

Preheat oven to 350°F. Combine the turkey, onion, rice, mint, egg, broth, salt, and pepper and sauté in olive oil until browned. In another pot, steam the cabbage until it is slightly soft. After the cabbage cools, cut off the bottom, peel off the leaves, and place them in a baking dish one by one. Spoon a helping of turkey mixture onto each leaf and then roll it up. Sprinkle with flaxseed and bake for 15–20 minutes. Makes 8 servings.

NUTRITION FACTS

Amount Per Serving: Calories 290 – Calories from Fat 100 – Total Fat 12 g
Saturated Fat 2.5 g – Cholesterol 70 mg – Sodium 130 mg – Total Carbohydrate 31 g
Dietary Fiber 6 g – Sugars 6 g – Protein 18 g – Calcium 10% DV

Rosemary Baked Chicken Breast

4 skinless, boneless chicken breasts
2 tablespoons minced garlic
3 tablespoons fresh rosemary or 4 tablespoons
    dried rosemary
2 tablespoon lemon juice
Salt and pepper to taste

Preheat the oven to 375°F. Put the chicken breasts in a baking dish and cover them with garlic, then sprinkle with rosemary, lemon juice, salt, and pepper. Bake uncovered for 25 minutes. Makes 4 servings.

NUTRITION FACTS

Amount Per Serving: Calories 140 – Calories from Fat 15 – Total Fat 1.5 g – Saturated Fat 0 g – Cholesterol 70 mg – Sodium 80 mg – Total Carbohydrate 2 g Dietary Fiber 0 g – Sugars 0 g – Protein 28 g – Calcium 2% DV

Savory Spinach and Salmon Salad

3 tablespoons orange juice
2 tablespoons low-sodium soy sauce
2 teaspoons minced fresh ginger
1 teaspoon raw honey
1½ teaspoons extra-virgin olive oil
4 (6-ounce) salmon filets
2 cups fresh spinach, washed
½ cup mandarin orange slices
⅓ cup chopped green onions (scallions)
2 hard-boiled eggs, sliced
¼ cup ground almonds mixed with
    1 tablespoon ground or milled flaxseed

In a small bowl, combine the orange juice, soy sauce, ginger, and honey. Whisk, gradually adding the olive oil, until well blended.

Grill, bake, or poach the salmon filets. Make a bed of spinach on each of four plates. Place salmon in the center of each one. Garnish each with mandarin orange slices, scallions, and eggs. Drizzle the orange–soy sauce dressing over the entire plate and sprinkle with almond-flaxseed mixture. Makes 4 servings.

NUTRITION FACTS

Amount Per Serving: Calories 370 – Calories from Fat 170 – Total Fat 19 g
Saturated Fat 3 g – Cholesterol 200 mg – Sodium 430 mg – Total Carbohydrate 10 g
Dietary Fiber 2 g – Sugars 6 g – Protein 40 g – Calcium 8% DV

Spicy Kale and Beans

2 cups dried black-eyed peas
1 bunch kale (about 2 pounds)
1 large onion, diced
1 tablespoon extra-virgin olive oil
2 tablespoons white vinegar
¼ teaspoon crushed red pepper (optional)
2 hard-boiled eggs, chopped

Soak black-eyed peas overnight. The next day place the drained peas in a large saucepan, cover with water, and bring to a boil over high heat. Boil for 3 minutes. Remove the pan from the heat, cover tightly, and let stand for 1 hour. Wash kale, remove large stem ends, and coarsely chop the leaves.

Sauté the onion in a large skillet. Add the kale and cook for about 5 minutes, until the leaves are wilted but still bright green. Stir in black-eyed peas, vinegar, and crushed red pepper until entire mixture bubbles with heat. Top with the eggs before serving. Makes 8 servings.

NUTRITION FACTS

Amount Per Serving: Calories 200 – Calories from Fat 35 – Total Fat 4 g – Saturated Fat 0.5 g – Cholesterol 55 mg – Sodium 480 mg – Total Carbohydrate 32 g Dietary Fiber 7 g – Sugars 1 g – Protein 11 g – Calcium 20% DV

Tossed Turkey Bacon and Spinach Salad

½ cup sliced almonds
1 tablespoon sesame seeds
1 tablespoon flaxseed
8 slices cooked turkey bacon, chopped
2 cups raw spinach, washed
4 scallions, chopped fine

Dressing
¼ cup extra-virgin olive oil
2 tablespoons Worcestershire sauce
2 teaspoons garlic paste or crushed garlic
4 tablespoons lemon juice
1 raw egg
¾ teaspoon salt
¾ teaspoon pepper

Preheat oven to 350°F. Roast almonds, sesame seeds, and flaxseed for 3–5 minutes. Set aside. Mix turkey bacon, spinach, and scallions in a small bowl. Put the dressing ingredients in a blender and blend until well mixed. Toss the salad with the dressing. Sprinkle with nut-seed mix just before serving. Makes 2 servings.

NUTRITION FACTS

Amount Per Serving: Calories 740 – Calories from Fat 560 – Total Fat 62 g
Saturated Fat 11 g – Cholesterol 160 mg – Sodium 2420 mg – Total Carbohydrate 19 g
Dietary Fiber 6 g – Sugars 5 g – Protein 28 g – Calcium 20% DV

Tuna Melt

1 (12-ounce) can albacore tuna in water
2 tablespoons plain low-fat yogurt
1 hard-boiled egg, chopped
1 tablespoon minced fresh parsley
Salt and pepper to taste
4 slices whole-grain bread
1 tomato, sliced
½ cup grated skim milk mozzarella

Drain tuna and mix with yogurt, egg, and parsley. Add salt and pepper. Toast the bread in the toaster or in a 300°F oven for 3–5 minutes; it should be crisp to the touch. Cover the bread generously with tuna mixture, then top with a tomato slice and grated cheese. Return to the toaster or oven and broil until the cheese melts. Makes 4 servings.

NUTRITION FACTS

Amount Per Serving: Calories 190 – Calories from Fat 60 – Total Fat 7 g – Saturated Fat 3 g – Cholesterol 80 mg – Sodium 410 mg – Total Carbohydrate 15 g Dietary Fiber 2 g – Sugars 4 g – Protein 19 g – Calcium 15% DV

Turkey and Asparagus Wraps

16 asparagus spears
⅓ cup plain low-fat yogurt
1 teaspoon lemon juice
1 teaspoon curry powder
Salt and pepper to taste
1 pound deli-style turkey breast, sliced

Wash, trim, and steam asparagus spears until tender. Set aside to cool. Mix yogurt, lemon juice, curry powder, salt, and pepper in a small bowl. Place 2 or 3 slices of turkey breast on a plate. Spread with the yogurt mixture. Put asparagus spears on one end and roll up. Secure with toothpick if necessary. Serve immediately or refrigerate. Makes 4 servings.

NUTRITION FACTS

Amount Per Serving: Calories 140 – Calories from Fat 15 – Total Fat 1.5 g – Saturated Fat 0 g – Cholesterol 50 mg – Sodium 1200 mg – Total Carbohydrate 10 g Dietary Fiber 2 g – Sugars 3 g – Protein 25 g – Calcium 6% DV

Turkey, Apple, and Spinach Pita

2 tablespoons extra-virgin olive oil
2 tablespoons lemon juice
½ pound cooked turkey, cut into chunks
1 teaspoon nutmeg, or to taste
Salt and pepper to taste
1 medium apple, cored and thinly sliced
2 pita bread rounds, separated
Fresh spinach, washed
½ cup plain low-fat yogurt

Heat olive oil in a skillet over medium heat. Stir in lemon juice. Mix in turkey; season with nutmeg and salt and pepper. Continue cooking until heated through.

Remove from heat. Stir in apple. Stuff the pitas with fresh spinach leaves and the turkey mixture. Drizzle with yogurt. Makes 4 servings.

NUTRITION FACTS

Amount Per Serving: Calories 420 – Calories from Fat 80 – Total Fat 9 g – Saturated Fat 2 g – Cholesterol 95 mg – Sodium 410 mg – Total Carbohydrate 40 g Dietary Fiber 2 g – Sugars 5 g – Protein 42 g – Calcium 15% DV

Veggie Burgers

1 medium onion, chopped very fine
1 medium bell pepper, chopped very fine
Extra-virgin olive oil
2 cups cooked fresh spinach, drained and
    chopped fine
1 cup Mashed Cauliflower (see recipe on
    page 165)
1 can black beans, drained
1 tablespoon garlic powder
1 egg, beaten well
2 pieces whole-grain toast, crumbled fine
Salt and pepper to taste

Sauté onion and bell pepper in olive oil until onion is translucent. When mixture has cooled, place it in a large bowl and add all other ingredients, mixing well. Form patties and place on cookie sheet. Chill for at least 2 hours before browning in olive oil in a skillet on top of the stove, or bake at 400°F for 30 minutes. Makes 4 servings.

NUTRITION FACTS

Amount Per Serving: Calories 170 – Calories from Fat 30 – Total Fat 3 g – Saturated
Fat 1 g – Cholesterol 55 mg – Sodium 190 mg – Total Carbohydrate 26 g
Dietary Fiber 7 g – Sugars 5 g – Protein 10 g – Calcium 8% DV

VEGETABLE DISHES

Asian Cabbage

2½ cups finely shredded cabbage
1 cup grated carrots
1 cup fresh spinach
2 tablespoons extra-virgin olive oil
1 teaspoon grated ginger root
Dash of Tabasco or hot sauce (optional)
Lemon juice
1 tablespoon toasted sesame seeds

Stir-fry the cabbage, carrots, and spinach in olive oil in a skillet or wok. Once the vegetables are tender, stir in the grated ginger root and hot sauce. Before serving, sprinkle with lemon juice. Put on a plate and top with toasted sesame seeds. Makes 6 servings.

NUTRITION FACTS

Amount Per Serving: Calories 60 – Calories from Fat 45 – Total Fat 5 g – Saturated Fat 0.5 g – Cholesterol 0 mg – Sodium 20 mg – Total Carbohydrate 4 g – Dietary Fiber 1 g Sugars 2 g – Protein 1 g – Calcium 4% DV

Baked Rutabaga

Note: The rutabaga is a root vegetable that looks very much like a turnip with yellow-orange flesh and ridges at its neck. Although this beta carotene–rich vegetable has been grown and marketed in our country for nearly 200 years, it remains an uncommon food in American dining. It's actually a great tasting vegetable with a delicate sweetness and flavor that hints of the light freshness of cabbage and turnip. With its easy preparation and versatility, great nutrition, and excellent flavor, the rutabaga can easily become an endearing family favorite.

2 or 3 medium-size rutabagas
4 apples
1 teaspoon olive oil
1 teaspoon salt
⅛ teaspoon white pepper
2 tablespoons Smart Balance

Preheat oven to 350°F. Peel rutabagas and apples and slice them ¼-inch thick. Use the olive oil to grease the casserole dish then sprinkle with salt and pepper and dot with butter. Bake for 25–30 minutes. Makes 8 servings.

NUTRITION FACTS

Amount Per Serving: Calories 110 – Calories from Fat 35 – Total Fat 3.5 g – Saturated Fat 2 g – Cholesterol 10 mg – Sodium 320 mg – Total Carbohydrate 19 g Dietary Fiber 5 g – Sugars 14 g – Protein 2 g – Calcium 8% DV

Beets and Brussels Sprouts

4 medium beets
10–12 Brussels sprouts
Extra-virgin olive oil
1 small white onion, peeled and sliced thin
3 tablespoons frozen orange juice concentrate
2 teaspoons grated ginger
Salt and pepper to taste

Boil beets for 45 minutes or until tender by touch with a fork; drain when done. Remove and discard the outer leaves of the Brussels sprouts and boil them in a separate pan for 5 minutes. Drain and cut in half. Put olive oil in skillet, sauté onion, and add beets and Brussels sprouts. Cook until warm, about 2–3 minutes, then stir in orange juice concentrate and ginger. Salt and pepper to taste. Makes 6 servings.

NUTRITION FACTS

Amount Per Serving: Calories 70 – Calories from Fat 15 – Total Fat 2 g – Saturated Fat 0 g – Cholesterol 0 mg – Sodium 55 mg – Total Carbohydrate 12 g Dietary Fiber 3 g – Sugars 7 g – Protein 2 g – Calcium 2% DV

Best Baked Beans

1 (16-ounce) can lima beans
⅓ cup frozen corn kernels
2 chopped tomatoes
½ cup grated Cheddar cheese
Salt and pepper to taste

Preheat the oven to 350°F. Combine all ingredients and bake for 30 minutes. Makes 4 servings.

NUTRITION FACTS

Amount Per Serving: Calories 230 – Calories from Fat 50 – Total Fat 5 g – Saturated Fat 3 g – Cholesterol 15 mg – Sodium 95 mg – Total Carbohydrate 32 g Dietary Fiber 10 g – Sugars 2 g – Protein 14 g – Calcium 15% DV

Broccoli and Cauliflower
in Lime Dressing

1 tablespoon low-sodium soy sauce
2 teaspoons raw honey
3 tablespoons fresh lime juice
1 cup broccoli florets
1 cup cauliflower florets
Salt and pepper to taste
Red pepper flakes (optional)

Mix soy sauce, honey, and lime juice. Set aside.

Boil broccoli and cauliflower for about 5 minutes, till they are tender yet firm. Drain and toss immediately with soy sauce–lime mixture. Season with salt and pepper to taste. Sprinkle with red pepper flakes if desired. Makes 4 servings.

NUTRITION FACTS

Amount Per Serving: Calories 30 – Calories from Fat 0 – Total Fat 0 g – Saturated Fat 0 g – Cholesterol 0 mg – Sodium 170 mg – Total Carbohydrate 7 g Dietary Fiber 1 g – Sugars 4 g – Protein 2 g – Calcium 2% DV

Cruciferous Couscous

1 cup minced broccoli
1 cup fresh spinach
1 cup minced cauliflower
2 tomatoes, cubed
2 tablespoons minced garlic
2 tablespoons extra-virgin olive oil
3 cups water
2 cups quick-cook couscous
2 tablespoons balsamic vinegar
Salt and pepper to taste

Preheat oven to 350°F. Mix broccoli, spinach, cauliflower, and tomatoes with garlic and 1 tablespoon of olive oil and place on a baking sheet. Bake for 15–20 minutes, until tender. In a pot, bring water and remaining tablespoon of olive oil to a boil, add couscous and return to a boil, then remove from heat and let stand for 5 minutes. Fluff with a fork and let cool. Place couscous on a plate and top with roasted vegetables. Drizzle with balsamic vinegar before serving. Makes 8 servings.

NUTRITION FACTS

Amount Per Serving: Calories 220 – Calories from Fat 35 – Total Fat 4 g – Saturated Fat 0.5 g – Cholesterol 0 mg – Sodium 20 mg – Total Carbohydrate 38 g Dietary Fiber 3 g – Sugars 2 g – Protein 6 g – Calcium 4% DV

Dressed-Up Asparagus

1 pound fresh asparagus
2 tablespoons extra-virgin olive oil
2 teaspoons lemon juice
Salt and pepper to taste
1½ tablespoons finely chopped almonds
1 tablespoon toasted flaxseed

Wash asparagus and trim ends. Steam for 3–5 minutes, until bright green and tender but crisp. While asparagus is steaming, mix together olive oil, lemon juice, salt, and pepper. In a separate bowl, mix the almonds and flaxseed. Drain asparagus and arrange on a serving platter. Drizzle with olive oil–lemon juice mix and then sprinkle with nut-seed mix. Serve immediately. Makes 4 servings.

NUTRITION FACTS

Amount Per Serving: Calories 120 – Calories from Fat 80 – Total Fat 9 g – Saturated Fat 1 g – Cholesterol 0 mg – Sodium 0 mg – Total Carbohydrate 6 g – Dietary Fiber 3 g Sugars 3 g – Protein 3 g – Calcium 4% DV

Easy Pickled Beets

4 (15-ounce) cans of beets
¼ cup xylitol (natural sugar substitute)
1 cup apple cider vinegar
½ cup orange juice

Drain beets. Mix sugar substitute, vinegar, and orange juice. Pour over beets and refrigerate overnight. Makes 8–10 servings.

NUTRITION FACTS

Amount Per Serving: Calories 60 – Calories from Fat 0 – Total Fat 0 g – Saturated Fat 0 g – Cholesterol 0 mg – Sodium 95 mg – Total Carbohydrate 13 g Dietary Fiber 2 g – Sugars 10 g – Protein 2 g – Calcium 2% DV

Green and Yellow Veggie Hash

2 small acorn squash, diced
2 grated carrots
½ green apple, diced
1 shallot, finely chopped
3 tablespoons extra-virgin olive oil
1 cup greens (kale, spinach, or turnip,
    collard, or mustard greens), cleaned, washed
    and shredded
1 tablespoon minced garlic
4 sprigs fresh sage
Salt and pepper to taste

Sauté the squash, carrots, green apple, and shallots in olive oil until tender. Mix in the greens, garlic, sage, salt, and pepper and continue cooking for 5 more minutes. Makes 6 servings.

NUTRITION FACTS

Amount Per Serving: Calories 140 – Calories from Fat 70 – Total Fat 7 g – Saturated Fat 1 g – Cholesterol 0 mg – Sodium 25 mg – Total Carbohydrate 20 g Dietary Fiber 3 g – Sugars 5 g – Protein 2 g – Calcium 6% DV

Grilled Asparagus with Sesame Seeds

4 tablespoons extra-virgin olive oil
1 pound fresh asparagus, trimmed and peeled
1 teaspoon salt
1 tablespoon sesame seeds

Drizzle the olive oil over the asparagus and turn spears until they are coated. Sprinkle with salt. Grill asparagus for 5 minutes on a hot grill, turning each minute or so. Remove and toss with sesame seeds. Makes 4 servings.

NUTRITION FACTS

Amount Per Serving: Calories 90 – Calories from Fat 70 – Total Fat 8 g – Saturated Fat 1 g – Cholesterol 0 mg – Sodium 0 mg – Total Carbohydrate 5 g – Dietary Fiber 3 g Sugars 2 g – Protein 3 g – Calcium 4% DV

Indian-Style Brussels Sprouts

2 tablespoons extra-virgin olive oil
1 teaspoon black or brown mustard seeds
2 teaspoons grated fresh ginger root
1 teaspoon ground coriander
½ teaspoon turmeric
½ teaspoon ground cardamom
⅛ teaspoon cayenne pepper
12 Brussels sprouts, cut in half
½ cup unsweetened organic apple juice
2 tablespoons fresh lemon juice
Salt and pepper to taste

Heat the olive oil in a skillet or saucepan. Add the mustard seeds and cook until they begin to pop. Stir in ginger, coriander, turmeric, cardamom, cayenne, and Brussels sprouts. Pour in the apple and lemon juices, add salt and pepper, then cover and simmer until tender, about 5 minutes. Makes 6 servings.

NUTRITION FACTS

Amount Per Serving: Calories 90 – Calories from Fat 45 – Total Fat 5 g – Saturated Fat 0.5 g – Cholesterol 0 mg – Sodium 20 mg – Total Carbohydrate 10 g Dietary Fiber 3 g – Sugars 4 g – Protein 3 g – Calcium 4% DV

Kale and Sauerkraut

1 bunch kale
1 can sauerkraut, drained

Steam kale leaves until tender but still green. Stir in one can of sauerkraut before serving.

NUTRITION FACTS

Amount Per Serving: Calories 30 – Calories from Fat 5 – Total Fat 0 g – Saturated Fat 0 g – Cholesterol 0 mg – Sodium 480 mg – Total Carbohydrate 7 g Dietary Fiber 3 g – Sugars 1 g – Protein 2 g – Calcium 8% DV

Lemon-Curry Cauliflower and Kale

1 teaspoon curry powder
2 teaspoons lemon zest
3 tablespoons lemon juice
1 bunch kale
1 head cauliflower
Salt and pepper to taste

Mix curry powder, lemon zest, and lemon juice. Set aside. Boil kale and cauliflower in a large pot of water with salt and pepper for 4–5 minutes, until tender. Drain and toss with lemon juice mixture. Makes 4 servings.

NUTRITION FACTS

Amount Per Serving: Calories 70 – Calories from Fat 5 – Total Fat 0.5 g – Saturated Fat 0 g – Cholesterol 0 mg – Sodium 70 mg – Total Carbohydrate 15 g Dietary Fiber 5 g – Sugars 4 g – Protein 5 g – Calcium 10% DV

Marinated Broccoli, Cucumber, and Tomato Salad

1 head of broccoli
2 medium cucumbers
1 cup cherry tomatoes, halved
¼ cup extra-virgin olive oil
⅛ cup lemon juice
¾ cup apple cider vinegar
3 tablespoons minced parsley
Salt and pepper to taste
¼ cup low-fat feta cheese
Fresh spinach

Cut the broccoli into florets and steam on top of the stove for 3 minutes; let cool. Chop the cucumber into bite-size pieces, toss with cherry tomatoes, and then add the cooled broccoli. In a small bowl, mix olive oil, lemon juice, vinegar, parsley, salt, and pepper. Pour the mixture over the vegetables. Place in refrigerator and chill overnight. Toss with feta cheese right before serving on a bed of spinach. Makes 8 servings.

NUTRITION FACTS

Amount Per Serving: Calories 110 – Calories from Fat 70 – Total Fat 8 g – Saturated Fat 1.5 g – Cholesterol 0 mg – Sodium 115 mg – Total Carbohydrate 6 g Dietary Fiber 2 g – Sugars 3 g – Protein 4 g – Calcium 6% DV

Mashed Cauliflower

1 medium head of cauliflower
Salt and pepper to taste
¼ cup skim milk
¼ cup instant low-carb mashed potatoes
1 teaspoon garlic paste or garlic powder
2 slices cooked turkey bacon, crumbled

Cut cauliflower into florets and steam with salt and pepper until very tender. Place in blender and add all ingredients except turkey bacon. Blend until smooth. Return to pot on stove to reheat if necessary. Garnish with crumbled turkey bacon. Makes 4 servings.

NUTRITION FACTS

Amount Per Serving: Calories 110 – Calories from Fat 40 – Total Fat 4.5 g
Saturated Fat 1.5 g – Cholesterol 15 mg – Sodium 380 mg – Total Carbohydrate 13 g
Dietary Fiber 4 g – Sugars 4 g – Protein 8 g – Calcium 6% DV

Roasted Beets

8 beets, peeled and quartered
3 tablespoons extra-virgin olive oil
1 teaspoon salt
1 teaspoon pepper

Preheat oven to 425°F. Place beets on a large baking pan and toss with oil, salt, and pepper. Bake for 1 hour and 30 minutes. Makes 6 servings.

NUTRITION FACTS

Amount Per Serving: Calories 110 – Calories from Fat 60 – Total Fat 7 g
Saturated Fat 1 g – Cholesterol 0 mg – Sodium 480 mg – Total Carbohydrate 11 g
Dietary Fiber 3 g – Sugars 7 g – Protein 2 g – Calcium 2% DV

Rutabagas and Nutmeg

4 large rutabagas
¼ teaspoon salt
Water
1 tablespoon extra-virgin olive oil
Black pepper
Dash of nutmeg

Peel rutabagas with a vegetable peeler and cut into chunks. Put them in a saucepan, add the salt, and cover with water. Bring to a boil. Turn heat down to medium and cook 12–15 minutes, or until fork tender. Drain, but save the cooking liquid.

Using a potato masher, coarsely mash the rutabagas in the saucepan, adding the cooking liquid as needed for moisture. Add olive oil, more salt if necessary, and pepper to taste. Transfer to a serving bowl and garnish with a dash of nutmeg. Makes 6 servings.

NUTRITION FACTS

Amount Per Serving: Calories 110 – Calories from Fat 25 – Total Fat 3 g – Saturated Fat 0 g – Cholesterol 0 mg – Sodium 150 mg – Total Carbohydrate 21 g Dietary Fiber 6 g – Sugars 14 g – Protein 3 g – Calcium 10% DV

Simple Greens and Garlic

Note: This recipe works well for kale, spinach, turnip greens, collard greens, or arugula.

    3 tablespoons extra-virgin olive oil
    1 onion, chopped
    3 cloves garlic, minced
    2 pounds greens, washed, dried, and
        shredded
    Salt and pepper

Heat olive oil over medium-high heat in a large frying pan. Add onion and garlic; cook and stir until soft. Stir in greens and cook until wilted. Salt and pepper to taste. Serve hot or warm. Makes 4 servings.

NUTRITION FACTS

Amount Per Serving: Calories 180 – Calories from Fat 100 – Total Fat 11 g
Saturated Fat 1.5 g – Cholesterol 0 mg – Sodium 45 mg – Total Carbohydrate 16 g
Dietary Fiber 9 g – Sugars 2 g – Protein 6 g – Calcium 35% DV

Skillet Broccoli or Asparagus with Sesame Seeds

2 large stalks fresh broccoli or
  12–14 asparagus spears
2 tablespoons extra-virgin olive oil
2 tablespoons sesame seeds
2 or 3 cloves garlic, peeled and sliced
Salt and pepper to taste

Wash broccoli and cut the florets into medium to large pieces. Peel the tough outer layer from the stems and slice the inner tender, juicy portion in half. Or, if using asparagus, wash the spears and trim off the ends. In a large skillet with a lid, heat the oil over high heat. Add sesame seeds and sauté, stirring until lightly toasted; be careful not to overcook, because they burn quickly. Also, keep the lid handy because the sesame seeds might start to pop. Add the broccoli (or asparagus) and garlic, and stir for a few seconds. Add salt and pepper to taste, and stir. Cover the skillet and remove from heat; let sit about 15 minutes. The broccoli (or asparagus) will retain its color and be tender and crisp. Makes 6 servings.

NUTRITION FACTS

Amount Per Serving: Calories 70 – Calories from Fat 50 – Total Fat 6 g – Saturated Fat 1 g – Cholesterol 0 mg – Sodium 0 mg – Total Carbohydrate 3 g – Dietary Fiber 1 g Sugars 1 g – Protein 1 g – Calcium 4% DV

Spinach and Feta Brown Rice

1 cup brown rice
1 cup fresh spinach leaves
2 teaspoons minced garlic
4 tablespoons low-fat feta cheese
Salt and pepper to taste

Cook the brown rice according to directions on the package, or bring to a boil 2 parts water to 1 part rice in a medium-sized pot, then cook on low for 30–45 minutes until the rice is soft. Before serving, add the spinach and garlic, stirring until the spinach wilts. Put on a plate and garnish with feta cheese. Makes 6 servings.

NUTRITION FACTS

Amount Per Serving: Calories 120 – Calories from Fat 15 – Total Fat 1.5 g
Saturated Fat 0.5 g – Cholesterol 0 mg – Sodium 70 mg – Total Carbohydrate 24 g
Dietary Fiber 1 g – Sugars 0 g – Protein 4 g – Calcium 2% DV

SALADS, SALAD DRESSINGS, AND SNACKS

Banana in Bark

1 tablespoon ground almonds
1 tablespoon ground or milled flaxseed
1 whole banana

Mix almonds and flaxseeds on a large plate. Peel banana and roll in mixture until fully covered. Either eat immediately or place on wax paper and put in refrigerator to chill before eating. Makes 1 serving.

NUTRITION FACTS

Amount Per Serving: Calories 200 – Calories from Fat 70 – Total Fat 7 g
Saturated Fat 0.5 g Cholesterol 0 mg – Sodium 0 mg – Total Carbohydrate 36 g
Dietary Fiber 6 g – Sugars 20 g – Protein 4 g Calcium 4% DV

Beet and Orange Salad

1 jar pickled beets
2 cans mandarin oranges in water, or 2 tanger-
    ines, peeled, sectioned, and seeded
½ cup orange juice
1 cup fresh spinach
¼ cup slivered almonds

Toss beets and mandarin orange or tangerine sections in orange juice. Chill for at least 1 hour. Serve on bed of spinach. Garnish with slivered almonds. Makes 4 servings.

NUTRITION FACTS

Amount Per Serving: Calories 150 – Calories from Fat 30 – Total Fat 3.5 g
Saturated Fat 0 g – Cholesterol 0 mg – Sodium 80 mg – Total Carbohydrate 28 g
Dietary Fiber 4 g – Sugars 22 g – Protein 4 g – Calcium 6% DV

Cabbage-Apple Salad

1 cup shredded cabbage
1 cup diced apple
1 cup chopped celery
¼ cup plain low-fat yogurt
2 tablespoons flaxseed

Mix all ingredients in a large bowl. Toss, chill, and serve.
Makes 6 servings.

NUTRITION FACTS
Amount Per Serving: Calories 45 – Calories from Fat 15 – Total Fat 2 g
Saturated Fat 0 g – Cholesterol 0 mg – Sodium 25 mg – Total Carbohydrate 7 g
Dietary Fiber 2 g – Sugars 4 g – Protein 2 g – Calcium 4% DV

Carrot and Orange Salad

1 cup grated carrots
½ teaspoon lemon juice
2 tablespoons frozen orange
   juice concentrate
1 tablespoon plain low-fat yogurt
1 (16-ounce) carton 1% milk fat cottage cheese
2 (5-ounce) cans mandarin oranges packed in
   water (not syrup), drained
Fresh spinach

Mix all ingredients in a large bowl except for 1 can of the mandarin oranges and spinach. Place salad on a bed of spinach for each serving. Garnish each serving with the remaining mandarin oranges. Makes 6 servings.

NUTRITION FACTS

Amount Per Serving: Calories 90 – Calories from Fat 10 – Total Fat 1 g
Saturated Fat 0.5 g – Cholesterol 5 mg – Sodium 350 mg – Total Carbohydrate 11 g
Dietary Fiber 2 g – Sugars 8 g – Protein 11 g – Calcium 10% DV

Chicken and Cold Rice Salad

2 cups cooked brown rice (you may use whole-
grain minute brown rice)
2½ cups cooked chicken, cubed
1 cup broccoli florets, steamed al dente
½ cup shredded almonds
2 tablespoons minced parsley
1 cup plain low-fat yogurt
Spinach
4 tangerines

Toss everything together in a large bowl except the
spinach and tangerines. Chill for at least 2 hours. Serve
on a bed of spinach and surround with tangerine slices.
Makes 10 servings.

NUTRITION FACTS

Amount Per Serving: Calories 170 – Calories from Fat 40 – Total Fat 4.5 g – Saturated
Fat 1 g – Cholesterol 30 mg – Sodium 70 mg – Total Carbohydrate 18 g
Dietary Fiber 3 g – Sugars 6 g – Protein 15 g – Calcium 10% DV

Celebration Salsa

4 ripe tomatoes, diced

4 scallions, chopped

1 large cucumber, minced

1 large orange, sectioned, seeded, and cut into
small pieces

1 tablespoon fresh cilantro, minced

2 tablespoons lemon juice

Salt to taste

Combine all ingredients in a large bowl. Refrigerate for at least 1 hour before serving to allow flavors to blend. This will keep in the refrigerator for 2–3 days. Makes 6 servings.

NUTRITION FACTS

Amount Per Serving: Calories 35 – Calories from Fat 5 – Total Fat 0 g
Saturated Fat 0 g – Cholesterol 0 mg – Sodium 10 mg – Total Carbohydrate 8 g
Dietary Fiber 2 g – Sugars 5 g – Protein 1 g – Calcium 4% DV

Creamy Coleslaw

4 cups shredded cabbage
1 cup grated carrots
1½ cups plain low-fat yogurt
1½ tablespoons finely chopped celery
1 teaspoon grated onion
3 tablespoons white vinegar
1 tablespoon raw honey
¾ teaspoon salt
Dash of pepper

Mix all ingredients in a large bowl and toss well. Refrigerate for at least 2 hours before serving. Makes 10 servings.

NUTRITION FACTS

Amount Per Serving: Calories 40 – Calories from Fat 5 – Total Fat 0.5 g – Total Carbohydrate 7 g – Dietary Fiber 1 g – Sugars 6 g – Protein 2 g – Calcium 8% DV

Cucumber and Yogurt Dressing

1 large cucumber
1 cup plain low-fat yogurt
1 tablespoon extra-virgin olive oil
½ teaspoon salt
½ teaspoon dill

Combine all ingredients in a blender and blend well. Refrigerate for at least 1 hour, then serve. This will keep in the refrigerator for 2 days. Makes 6 servings.

NUTRITION FACTS

Amount Per Serving: Calories 50 – Calories from Fat 25 – Total Fat 3 g – Saturated Fat 0.5 g – Cholesterol 0 mg – Sodium 220 mg – Total Carbohydrate 4 g – Dietary Fiber 0 g – Sugars 4 g – Protein 2 g – Calcium 8% DV

Favorite Chicken Salad

4 (4-ounce) chicken breasts, boiled and diced
4 hard-boiled eggs, sliced
1 cup sliced celery
1 medium apple, chopped
½ cup plain low-fat yogurt
2 tablespoons lemon juice
1 teaspoon salt
1 teaspoon pepper
Fresh spinach
½ cup finely chopped almonds

Combine all ingredients except almonds. Place in refrigerator for at least 4 hours. Serve over fresh spinach and top with chopped almonds. Makes 8 servings.

NUTRITION FACTS

Amount Per Serving: Calories 190 – Calories from Fat 70 – Total Fat 8 g – Saturated Fat 2 g – Cholesterol 155 mg – Sodium 390 mg – Total Carbohydrate 6 g Dietary Fiber 2 g – Sugars 4 g – Protein 23 g – Calcium 8% DV

Flaxseed and Fruit Smoothie

1 cup skim milk
1 cup frozen berries
1 banana
1 cup plain low-fat yogurt
1 tablespoon flaxseed oil
1 tablespoon ground flaxseed

Combine all ingredients except flaxseed in blender. Blend well. Pour into large glass and stir in flaxseed. Makes 1 serving.

NUTRITION FACTS

Amount Per Serving: Calories 580 – Calories from Fat 200 – Total Fat 23 g – Saturated Fat 4 g – Cholesterol 20 mg – Sodium 310 mg – Total Carbohydrate 78 g Dietary Fiber 7 g – Sugars 58 g – Protein 25 g – Calcium 70% DV

Ginger-Lime Dressing

1 cup low-sodium soy sauce
2 tablespoons minced garlic
2 tablespoons grated fresh ginger root
2 teaspoons sesame oil
⅓ cup fresh lime juice
¼ cup rice vinegar

Place all ingredients in blender. Blend until well mixed.
Chill for at least 1 hour, then serve. Makes 6 servings.

NUTRITION FACTS

Amount Per Serving: Calories 50 – Calories from Fat 15 – Total Fat 1.5 g – Saturated
Fat 0 g – Cholesterol 0 mg – Sodium 1600 mg – Total Carbohydrate 7 g
Dietary Fiber 1 g – Sugars 1 g – Protein 3 g – Calcium 2% DV

Grapefruit and Avocado Salad

2 whole Ruby Red grapefruits
1 medium ripe avocado
3 tablespoons orange juice
2 tablespoons plain low-fat yogurt
1 teaspoon raw honey
1 teaspoon poppy seeds
Fresh spinach

Peel, section, and seed grapefruit. Peel avocado and slice lengthwise. Mix orange juice, yogurt, and honey, whisking until well blended. Stir in poppy seeds. Arrange grapefruit and avocado together on bed of spinach. Drizzle with orange–poppy seed dressing. Makes 4 servings.

NUTRITION FACTS

Amount Per Serving: Calories 130 – Calories from Fat 60 – Total Fat 6 g – Saturated Fat 1 g – Cholesterol 0 mg – Sodium 30 mg – Total Carbohydrate 19 g Dietary Fiber 3 g – Sugars 3 g – Protein 3 g – Calcium 6% DV

Grated Beet Salad

2 tablespoons lemon juice
¾ cup orange juice
2 pounds fresh beets, peeled and grated
Salt and pepper to taste
⅓ cup chopped fresh parsley

Add lemon juice to orange juice and stir. Toss in grated beets. Add salt and pepper. Chill at least 1 hour and toss in parsley before serving. Makes 8 servings.

NUTRITION FACTS

Amount Per Serving: Calories 60 – Calories from Fat 0 – Total Fat 0 g – Saturated Fat 0 g – Cholesterol 0 mg – Sodium 90 mg – Total Carbohydrate 14 g Dietary Fiber 2 g – Sugars 11 g – Protein 2 g – Calcium 2% – DV

Marinated Cucumber, Radishes, and Onion Salad

½ cup rice wine vinegar
¼ cup extra-virgin olive oil
1 tablespoon chopped fresh dill or
  1 teaspoon dried dill
1 large cucumber, sliced thin
½ cup sliced radishes
1 medium red onion, sliced thin

Mix vinegar, olive oil, and dill in a large bowl. Add cucumber, radishes, and onion. Toss to coat. Refrigerate at least 3 hours, stirring at least once an hour to allow flavors to meld. Makes 8 servings.

NUTRITION FACTS

Amount Per Serving: Calories 80 – Calories from Fat 60 – Total Fat 7 g – Saturated Fat 1 g – Cholesterol 0 mg – Sodium 0 mg – Total Carbohydrate 4 g Dietary Fiber 1 g – Sugars 2 g – Protein 0 g – Calcium 2% DV

Not Your Ordinary Tuna Salad

1 large (12-ounce) can white albacore tuna in
    water
1 red pepper, chopped fine
1 yellow pepper, chopped fine
¼ cup grated green apple
⅓ cup shredded fresh cabbage
2 tablespoons plain low-fat yogurt
½ teaspoon lemon juice
½ teaspoon rice wine vinegar
Salt and pepper to taste

Mix all ingredients together in a large bowl. Chill for at
least 1 hour before serving. Makes 4 servings.

NUTRITION FACTS

Amount Per Serving: Calories 70 – Calories from Fat 15 – Total Fat 1.5 g – Saturated
Fat 0 g – Cholesterol 20 mg – Sodium 170 mg – Total Carbohydrate 4 g
Dietary Fiber 1 g – Sugars 3 g – Protein 11 g – Calcium 2% DV

Sauerkraut Salad

1 (16-ounce) can sauerkraut
4 cups chopped onion
1 cup sliced pimento
4 cups chopped celery
2 cups chopped broccoli
½ cup white vinegar
Salt and pepper to taste

Toss all ingredients together in a very large bowl and refrigerate overnight. This will keep in the refrigerator for up to a week. Makes 12 servings.

NUTRITION FACTS

Amount Per Serving: Calories 40 – Calories from Fat 0 – Total Fat 0 g – Saturated Fat 0 g – Cholesterol 0 mg – Sodium 290 mg – Total Carbohydrate 9 g Dietary Fiber 3 g – Sugars 4 g – Protein 2 g – Calcium 4% DV

Simple Cheese Toast

Organic nonstick cooking spray
6 slices whole-grain bread
Extra-virgin olive oil
2 tomatoes, sliced
3 tablespoons grated Cheddar cheese
3 tablespoons grated skim milk mozzarella
    cheese

Preheat oven to 300°F. Arrange bread on flat baking sheet that you have sprayed with organic nonstick baking spray. Brush bread tops with olive oil. Toast in oven for 5–7 minutes or until bread is firm and crisp to the touch. Remove and top each piece of bread with a slice of tomato; sprinkle with cheese. Return bread to oven and broil until cheese melts and is bubbly, usually less than 3 minutes. Makes 6 servings.

NUTRITION FACTS

Amount Per Serving: Calories 110 – Calories from Fat 30 – Total Fat 3.5 g
Saturated Fat 1.5 g – Cholesterol 5 mg – Sodium 180 mg – Total Carbohydrate 14 g
Dietary Fiber 2 g – Sugars 4 g – Protein 6 g – Calcium 6% DV

Spinach Salad with
Beets in Cottage Cheese

4 medium beets
¼ cup extra-virgin olive oil
3 tablespoons lemon juice
½ teaspoon raw honey
¼ teaspoon dry mustard
Salt and pepper to taste
½ cup 1% milk fat cottage cheese
2 tablespoons milled flaxseed
2 cups fresh spinach

Boil beets until tender and let cool. While beets are cooling, mix olive oil, lemon juice, raw honey, dry mustard, and salt and pepper. Peel and slice beets into strips, then mix with cottage cheese and flaxseed. Place on bed of spinach. Drizzle the salad with the dressing mixture. Makes 4 servings.

NUTRITION FACTS

Amount Per Serving: Calories 210 – Calories from Fat 150 – Total Fat 16 g
Saturated Fat 2.5 g – Cholesterol 0 mg – Sodium 190 mg – Total Carbohydrate 12 g
Dietary Fiber 4 g – Sugars 7 g – Protein 6 g – Calcium 6% DV

Yogurt and Fruit Parfait

⅓ cup ground almonds
2 tablespoons ground or milled flaxseed
1 cup plain low-fat yogurt
¾ cup berries
Raw honey (optional)

In small bowl, mix almonds with flaxseed. In parfait glass, alternately layer yogurt, berries, and almond-flaxseed mixture. If desired, drizzle a small amount of honey on top. Makes 1 serving.

NUTRITION FACTS

Amount Per Serving: Calories 480 – Calories from Fat 240 – Total Fat 27 g
Saturated Fat 4.5 g – Cholesterol 15 mg – Sodium 180 mg – Total Carbohydrate 47 g
Dietary Fiber 8 g – Sugars 25 g – Protein 23 g – Calcium 60% DV

APPENDIX A

Journal and Food Diary

M any of the people who have been successful on the plan report that they made the best progress when they monitored themselves by writing things down. The following can be used as your daily tracking tool. Make thirty copies, one for each day of the month, and fill in every day.

Date: _____

Weight: _____

Waistline measurement
(first week of each month only): _____

A. Circle the reply that best fits for each of the following categories.
   1. Sleep:
      - a full eight hours

- sporadically waking up through the night with hot flashes
- not sleeping at all

2. Energy:
   - rested and ready to go
   - sluggish and slow
   - fatigued; wish I could go back to bed

3. Mood:
   - extremely upbeat
   - positive
   - indifferent
   - irritable and moody
   - depressed

4. Libido, sex drive:
   - always strong
   - very high right now
   - not great now but never good in the morning
   - neutral or indifferent
   - very low
   - comatose

5. Body image:
   - feel good about my body size and shape
   - feel positive about some weight loss and change in body shape
   - feel just okay
   - feel frustrated

B. Check the symptoms of hormone imbalance that you are experiencing today.
   1. Women:
      ❑ Weight gain   ❑ Mood swings   ❑ Hot flashes

❑ Night sweats ❑ Fatigue ❑ Headaches
❑ Depression ❑ Anxiety ❑ Nervousness
❑ Irritability ❑ Teariness ❑ Memory lapse
❑ Premature aging ❑ Vaginal dryness
❑ Heavy menses ❑ Bleeding changes
❑ Incontinence ❑ Fibrocystic breasts
❑ Decreased sex drive ❑ Tender breasts
❑ Osteoporosis ❑ Water retention

2. Premenopausal or perimenopausal women:
   • My last menstrual cycle started on _____ (date).
   • I am currently menstruating; this is the _____ day of my cycle.

3. Men:
   ❑ Weight gain ❑ Burned-out feeling
   ❑ Abdominal fat ❑ Prostate problems
   ❑ Decreased mental clarity ❑ Decreased sex drive
   ❑ Increased urinary urge ❑ Decreased strength
   ❑ Decreased stamina ❑ Difficulty sleeping
   ❑ Decreased urine flow ❑ Irritability
   ❑ Depression ❑ Erectile dysfunction
   ❑ Hot flashes ❑ Night sweats ❑ Poor concentration

C. Stress Level
   1. On a scale of 0–10 (0 = no stress; 10 = high stress), my stress level is _____.

D. Exercise
   1. Last week I exercised _____ times per week for an average of _____ minutes each time.
   2. Describe the activity or activities: _____
   _____

E. Outlook

1. In addition to being grateful for making progress toward losing my unwanted belly fat, I am thankful for (list three things): _____

_____

_____

Your Belly Flat Food Diary

Most nutritionists and dietitians agree that keeping a food diary is critical to weight loss success. Keeping a thirty-day Food Diary will help you make hormone-healthy eating an easy habit to keep. It will also help you better identify when, where, how and with whom all your good intentions go by the wayside to the detriment of your waist size.

Here are a three helpful hints:

• **Write everything down.**
  Keep your diary with you all day. Write down every mouthful, even gum.

• **Tell the truth.**
  The only thing you have to gain by cheating on these forms is more weight.

• **Do it now.**
  Don't depend on your memory at the end of the day. Record everything you eat and drink as soon as it is consumed.

Daily Food Diary

Date:_____

	Time	What Did You Eat? Drink?	How Much?	Where?	With Whom?	What Were You Doing?	What Was Your Mood?
Breakfast							
Snack							
Lunch							
Snack							
Dinner							

Belly-Blasting Food Checklist

Food Group	Recommended Servings/Day	# of Servings You Had
Cruciferous Vegetables	2–3	
Citrus Fruits	1	
Insoluble Fiber	2	
Lignans	2–3 tablespoons	
Protein	3	
Calcium	2	
Fruit (other than citrus)	1	
Water	8–10 glasses	

Don't Forget to Supplement Your Weight Loss Success

Supplement	Recommended Dosage	What You Took	What Time
Bio-identical Progesterone Cream	• Women who are menstruating: twice daily from day 8–26 of your cycle • Women who are no longer menstruating or who are perimenopausal: twice daily for 25 days, then take 5 days off • Women also on bio-identical estrogen: twice daily, every day • Men: twice daily for 25 days then 5 days off		
Calcium D-Glucarate	1,000 mg twice daily		
DIM	Women should take 200 mg/day; men 400 mg/day		
B-Complex Vitamin	1 per day		
Vitamin E	400 IU per day		
Calcium-Magnesium Supplement	1,500 mg of calcium and 750 mg of magnesium		
7-Keto DHEA	100 mg each morning		
Chitosan	750 mg to 1 g three times a day; take with meals		

How Did You Take Care of You Today? Did You . . .

Activity	Doing What?	What Time?	How Long?	With Whom?
Consciously Take Time To De-Stress				
Exercise				
Laugh				
Sleep				

APPENDIX B

How to Reduce the Estrogens
in Your Environment

The following list can help you to take action to reduce the effect of environmental estrogens in your life:

- Because some plastics shed xenohormones when heated, assume that they all do, and protect yourself accordingly. Don't drink hot beverages from plastic cups and don't drink water from a plastic bottle that has been left in the sun or in a hot car.
- Don't microwave your food or drinks in plastic containers; avoid using plastic wrap to cover food in the microwave.
- Get a good-quality water filter for your home. Drink and cook with filtered water.

- When possible, eat only organic, hormone-free meat and dairy products.
- Eat organic produce, which has not been sprayed with pesticides.
- Wash all produce to rid it of any type of chemical residue or pesticides.
- Throw away all pesticides, herbicides, and fungicides.
- Never tent your house and fumigate it with pesticides.
- Research and use organic approaches and products for home gardening and pest control.
- Check product labels for the following chemicals: aliphatic hydrocarbons (n-hexane), halogenated hydrocarbons (carbon tetrachloride, trichlorethylene), alcohols (methanol, ethanol), cyclic hydrocarbons (cyclohexane), esters (ethyl acetate), ethers (ethyl ether), nitrohydrocarbons (ethyl nitrate), ketones (acetone, methylethylketone), glycols (ethylene glycol), aromatic hydrocarbons (benzene), and aldehydes (acetaldehyde). Do not buy products, or throw away those you already have, if these chemicals are present.
- Check your cosmetics for toxic ingredients and throw them away. Most health food stores now stock a variety of organic cosmetics and even natural hair dyes.
- Don't use fabric softeners.
- Exchange your perfumes and air fresheners for natural aromatic oils and fresh scents from your garden.
- Because most spermicidal products contain petrochemicals, avoid using lubricated condoms or vaginal gels.
- New homes or offices filled with new carpet, fiberboard,

new paint, and glues can give off a wide variety of toxic fumes. Consider flushing the toxins out of the air with a portable air filter prior to moving in.

- Never use synthetic hormone replacement.
- Evaluate your options for birth control and, whenever possible, find an alternative to birth control pills. If your personal choice is to use birth control pills for contraception, use for the shortest term possible.

ABOUT THE AUTHORS

C.W. Randolph, Jr., M.D., is an internationally recognized medical expert in the field of bio-identical hormone replacement, who has successfully treated thousands of women and men with hormone imbalances for more than a decade. He is a board-certified obstetrician and gynecologist who practiced as a compounding pharmacist before returning to medical school.

Dr. Randolph is also the co-founder of The Natural Hormone Institute of America, a Diplomate of the American Board of Holistic Medicine, and a member of The International Academy of Compounding Pharmacists.

He continues to be a frequent speaker for medical and women's organizations across the country and is also the coauthor of the best selling book, *From Hormone Hell to Hormone Well*.

Go to http://hormonewell.com/intertview.html to see Dr. Randolph's interview on the *CBS Early Show*.

For more than two decades, **Genie James** has been nationally acknowledged as a change-agent in women's health. In 2004, she co-founded The Natural Hormone Institute of America with C.W. Randolph, Jr., M.D., in order to create a vehicle for getting the word out about the safety and efficacy of bio-identical hormone therapies.

Genie also serves as the executive director of Women Evolving, LLC, an organization dedicated to educating women how to use their *choice, voice* and *financial power* to enhance their personal healthcare while, also, positively impacting our nation ' s overall healthcare delivery system.

In addition to coauthoring *From Hormone Hell to Hormone Well* and *From Belly Fat to Belly Flat* with Dr. Randolph, Genie is the author of *Making Managed Care Work* and *Winning in the Women's Healthcare Marketplace*.

APPENDIX C

Resources

Please note: The contact information listed in this section is current as of the publication of this book.

Hormone Health

The Natural Hormone Institute of America

When Genie James and I cofounded The Natural Hormone Institute of America in 2003, we had two goals in mind. The first was to create a vehicle to educate both the medical community and healthcare consumers about the safety and efficacy of bio-identical hormone therapies. Our second goal was to make my over-the-counter bio-identical progesterone cream and other products more widely available, committing a percentage of website profits to support medical research in the field of bio-identical hormone replacement.

To date, I have been overwhelmed by the positive response of many of my physician peers, as well as interested and educated healthcare consumers. I am grateful that The Natural Hormone Institute of America is meeting a very real need.

For more information regarding bio-identical hormone replacement, to discuss scheduling a personal consultation or to purchase the products recommended in this book, go to my interactive website www.hormonewell.com, or contact our office by telephone at 904-694-0039.

Over-the-Counter Progesterone Creams

You can purchase bio-identical progesterone creams in most health foods stores. The good news is that these creams are available; the bad news is that some products are better than others. The reason for this discrepancy: there is no regulatory body that oversees the production or standardization of product manufacturing for so-called "natural" products. What this means to the average consumer is that there is great variation among the many OTC progesterone creams on the market today.

While I cannot reveal the exact formula for my Natural Balance Cream, I can outline some of the critical variables that define its excellence and efficacy:

- *Dr. Randolph's Natural Balance Cream is a bio-identical formulation of progesterone.* This means that the molecules of progesterone suspended in the cream have exactly the same molecular structure as those produced by the human body. The body recognizes, receives, and utilizes these molecules. The parent molecule for progesterone comes from a substance known as *diosgenin,* which is found in soy or Mexican wild yam. Many products on the market today containing soy or Mexican wild yam claim to be a "natural progesterone"; however, until the diosgenin is converted from its original molecular structure, the body will not recognize it. Consequently, soy or Mexican wild yam in the raw state will not generate the same clinical response.

- *My Natural Balance Cream contains the maximum concentration of human- identical progesterone that can be mixed in an over-the-counter product.* Some creams have a small amount of progesterone in their mix, but not enough to generate a consistent and positive patient response.
- The progesterone I use in my formula meets the United States Pharmacopoeia gold standards for quality and purity. In addition, the lab I use to compound my cream operates under strict guidelines approved by the National Association of Compounding Pharmacists. This is *not* required by law, so not all product manufacturers go to the trouble or expense.
- *The progesterone molecule in my cream is encased within a liposomal delivery system.* This is critical because, as the many layers of the oily globule of liposome melt away like a snowball, the hormones are dispersed continuously through the skin for up to twelve hours. This means that the underlying issue of hormonal imbalance is eliminated, hormonal balance is restored and my patients have continuous relief of their symptoms throughout the day. In contrast, many over-the-counter progesterone creams are not formulated for sustained release. All the progesterone in these creams is immediately absorbed through

the skin, resulting in a quick spike in progesterone levels
and a temporary versus constant relief of symptoms.

There are several other over-the-counter creams that I have
reviewed for quality and truth in advertising. These include:

Arbonne International
PhytoProlief and Prolief Natural Balancing Creams
P.O. Box 2488
Laguna Hills, California
(800) ARBONNE or www.arbonne.com

Emerita
Pro-Gest progesterone cream
621 SW Alder, Suite 900
Portland, Oregon 97205
(800) 648-8211 or www.progest.com

The Health and Science Research Institute
Serenity for Women Natural Progesterone Cream
661 Beville Road, Suite 101
Daytona Beach, Florida 32119
(888) 222-1415 or www.health-science.com

HM Enterprises
Happy PMS
2622 Bailey Drive
Norcross, Georgia 30071
(800) 742-4773 or www.hmenterprises.com

Life-flo Health Care Products
ProgestaCare Cream
8146 N. 23rd Avenue, Suite E
Phoenix, Arizona 85021
(888) 999-7440 or www.sheld.com/lifeflo

Products of Nature
Natural Woman Progesterone Cream
2842 Main Street
Glastonbury, CT 06073
(800) 639-2499 or www.pronature.com

Restored Balance, Inc.
Restored Balance Premenstrual Menopausal Solutions Cream
42 Meadowbridge Drive
Cartersville, Georgia 30120
(800) 865-7499 or www.restoredbalanceusa.com

There are many other progesterone creams on the market today that I have not reviewed which may also contain bio-identical progesterone. If you have any doubt or concerns regarding any bio-identical progesterone product, call the company and ask how many milligrams of progesterone per ounce the cream contains.

Testing Hormone Levels

If you have not found relief from your symptoms from using a progesterone cream, this can be regarded as a signal that your hormone levels have begun to fluctuate. At this time, a saliva test or capillary blood spot testing may be an appropriate next step to evaluate the current ratio of all three sex hormones.

On my website, I offer a viable option for those women or men who believe or have evidence that their hormone balance has shifted and requires treatment. You can go to www.hormonewell.com/hormoneconsultation.html to learn more about how you can obtain a comprehensive hormone level profile via a saliva test or schedule a one-on-one telephone consultation with me or one of my personally trained nurse practitioners.

ZRT Laboratory's state-of-the-art saliva and capillary blood spot testing technology allows for accurate measurement of a broad array of hormones and detection of existing hormone imbalance.

1. *Saliva Testing*

Convenient home collection, accurate, and inexpensive, saliva testing provides a true picture of the bioavailable levels of steroid hormones.

2. *Capillary Blood Spot Testing*

Capillary blood spot testing offers an easy, finger-stick alternative to blood draws in the doctor's office.

3. *Combination Saliva and Capillary Blood Spot*

Combines both saliva and capillary blood spot test materials in an all-in-one test kit for easy home collection of the major hormone groups—reproductive, adrenal, and thyroid—on the same day at the optimal time.

Dr. David Zava, the founder of ZRT Laboratory, is also the coauthor with John R. Lee, M.D., of *What Your Doctor May Not Tell You About Breast Cancer.*

To find out more information, contact:

ZRT Laboratory
8605 SW Creekside Place
Beaverton, OR 97008
Phone: 503-466-2445
Fax: 503-466-1636
24-Hour Hotline: 503-466-9166
Website: www.zrtlab.com

Locating a Physician

There are two resources that I recommend if you are looking for a physician in your area who is knowledgeable about bio-identical hormone replacement. The first is the Women In Balance website, www.womeninbalance.org. The second is your local compounding pharmacist. If you need help finding a compounding pharmacy in your area, contact one of the two organizations listed below.

The International Academy of Compounding Pharmacists (IACP)
P.O. Box 1365
Sugar Land, TX 77487
Phone: 281-933-8400
Fax: 281-495-0602
Website: www.iacprx.org

IACP was established in 1991 as Professionals and Patients for Customized Care (P2C2). In 1996, P2C2 changed its name to IACP in an effort to broaden its scope and recognize changes in the profession. Today, the IACP has more than 1,800 members internationally, serving pharmacists, physicians, students, and patients.

Professional Compounding Centers of America (PCCA)
9901 South Wilcrest Drive
Houston, TX 77099
Phone: 877-798-3224
Fax: 877-765-1422
Website: www.pccarx.com

PCCA provides independent pharmacists with a complete support system from compounding unique dosage forms. Founded in 1981, PCCA has more than 3,000 pharmacist members located throughout the United States, Canada, Australia, Europe, and New Zealand. On an average, PCCA's consulting department answers more than 500 calls per day, providing members with comprehensive technical support.

"Belly Flat" Foods and Products

Organic Foods

Grocery Stores

Because of growing consumer demand, almost every grocery store in the nation stocks some organic foods. Still, my hat is off to two companies that over the last decade have taken the lead. They are:

Whole Foods Market: Founded in 1980 as one small store

in Austin, Texas, Whole Foods Market is now the world's leading retailer of natural and organic foods, with 197 stores in North America and the United Kingdom. To find a Whole Foods Market near you, go to www.wholefoodsmarket.com.

Wild Oats: In July 2007 it was announced that Wild Oats, another pioneer would merge with Whole Foods Market. Prior to the merger, Wild Oats operated 110 natural foods stores in 24 states and British Columbia, Canada. The Company's markets also include: Wild Oats Marketplace, Henry's Farmers Market, Sun Harvest and Capers Community Markets. At the time of this printing, Wild Oats website was still operational: www.wildoats.com.

Websites

Many people initially complain that buying organic is too expensive. Yes, organic foods can be pricey if you just shop in your supermarket, but you probably have a lot more choices for organic food in your community than you realize. All it takes is a little research to find out.

To find a source of organic foods near you or to order online, check out the following websites: www.organicfood.com, www.organicconsumer.org, www.eatwell.com, and www. diamondorganics.com. Also, local farmer's markets can be a great source for organic foods, often at lower prices than you will pay in the supermarket or health food store.

Favorite Brands

Vitamins and Supplements

When I opened my first Natural Medicine Store, I stocked the shelves with natural products from a variety of manufacturers. It was not long before the difference in my patients' and customers' responses signaled to me that not all product manufacturers could be trusted. According to a recent survey of nearly 1,000 supplements conducted by ConsumerLab.com, a product-certification company, one out of four supplements has quality problems, such as contamination or a failure to include an ingredient listed on the label.

As I became aware of the discrepancy between manufacturers, I drew on my professional training and experience as a compounding pharmacist to establish criteria that would insure that any product in my shop and on my website was safe and effective.

My criterion for my private-label products was and is simple yet non-negotiable: **quality and truth in labeling.** This means that for my own private-labeled line, as well as other natural health product lines that I carry, I require stringent guidelines for their manufacturing process. These guidelines include:

- Raw materials testing
- Potency testing
- Product traceability
- Purity testing
- Product freshness
- Microbiology testing

The bottom line is truth in packaging. People have the

right to know what they are putting in their bodies and they deserve to get the amount of active ingredient they are paying for.

To order Dr. Randolph's products online, go to www. hormonewell.com/shop_online.htm.

Life Extension is a highly reputable source for vitamins and supplements. This company's manufacturing standards ensure exceptional purity and quality. For Life Extension members purchasing products, the company provides access to a toll-free phone line where members can speak with holistic health advisors and medical doctors about their individual health concerns. In addition to its natural product offerings, Life Extension publishes a fantastic monthly magazine. For more information on Life Extension, go to www.lef.org or call 1-800-226-2370.

Whole Grains

Just because a bread, cereal, or pasta product is brown in color, don't assume that it is a whole-grain product. Check the ingredient list for the words "whole grain" or "whole wheat" to decide if they are made from a whole grain. Some foods are made from a mixture of whole and refined grains.

Some grain products contain significant amounts of bran. Bran provides fiber, which is important for health. However, products with added bran or bran alone (e.g., oat bran) are not necessarily whole-grain products.

On their website, www.wholegrainlife.com, General Mills offers excellent information regarding "What Is a Whole Grain?" and "How to Find a Whole Grain Product." The good news is that General Mills products are readily available in every grocery store across the nation.

Kashi (www.kashi.com) is another of one of my favorite whole-grain brands. I particularly love the Company's logo: "7 whole grains on a mission." I stock Kashi products in both of my Natural Medicine Stores, but they are also available on the health food or organic food aisle in almost any grocery store.

Another brand to check out is Food For Life (www.foodfor life.com). I am a huge fan of their organic sprouted whole-grain pastas and breads. Again, I stock Food for Life products in my Natural Medicine Store, but to find out where you can buy them, check out the website's built-in store finder.

Organic Housecleaning Products

Remember that it is important to decrease your exposure to environmental estrogens, or xenoestrogens. I recommend using organic housecleaning products when at all possible. Two good sources for online purchasing are www.heathers naturals.com and www.organiccleaning.com.

Safe Cosmetics

I urge you to make sure that your cosmetics are safe. Many are not. The Campaign for Safe Cosmetics is a coalition of public health, educational, religious, labor, women's, environmental, and consumer groups. The coalition's goal is to protect consumer health by requiring the health and beauty industry to phase out the use of chemicals linked to cancer, birth defects, and other health problems, and replace them with safer alternatives.

The Safe Cosmetics Campaign began in 2002 with the release of a report, Not Too Pretty: Phthalates, Beauty Products and the FDA. For the report, environmental and public health groups contracted with a laboratory to test seventy-two name-brand, off-the-shelf beauty products for the presence of phthalates, a family of industrial chemicals linked to permanent birth defects in the male reproductive system.

You can find a listing of who has pledged not to use harmful chemicals and to implement substitution plans that replace hazardous materials with safer alternatives in every market they serve on the Safe Cosmetics Campaign website: www.safecosmetics.org/companies/signers.cfm. Several major cosmetics companies, including OPI, Avon, Estee Lauder, L'Oreal, Revlon, Proctor & Gamble, and Unilever have thus far refused to sign the Compact for Safe Cosmetics.

The good news is that safe cosmetics are readily available. My coauthor Genie James's favorite source for safe or "green" make up and hair color is The Body Shop. Marketing Week has reported that The Body Shop was voted the Top Green Brand in the United Kingdom and the eighth greenest brand in the United States. These findings are according to the recent 2007 Image Power Green Brands Survey and Marketing Week/ Brand Index Online Survey. You can purchase The Body Shop products online, www.thebodyshop.com, or just head out to your nearest mall.

Recently Genie also discovered a delightful website where you can purchase safe cosmetics online. Check out www.themomspa.com.

Water Bottles

As stated in earlier chapters, you should be drinking a lot of water, but please beware of plastic water bottles. Plastics made from polycarbonate resin can leach bisphenol-A (BPA), a potent hormone disruptor. BPA, a chemical found in epoxy resin and polycarbonate plastics, may impair the reproductive organs and have adverse effects on tumors, breast tissue development, and prostate development by reducing sperm count.

BPA can leach into water bottles through normal wear and tear and exposure to heat and cleaning agents. This includes leaving your plastic water bottle in your car during errands, in your backpack during hikes, and running it through your dishwasher or using harsh detergents. What's more, a 2003 study conducted by the University of Missouri published in the journal, Environmental Health Perspectives, found that detectable levels of BPA leached into liquids at room temperature. This means just having your plastic water bottle sitting on your desk can be potentially harmful. The best thing to do is to avoid plastic altogether. (Side note: Baby bottles made from polycarbonate plastics have quietly disappeared from the market despite industry assurances that polycarbonate plastics are safe.)

There are two approaches to take to avoid exposure to BPA. First, if you are active and take water with you, switch to a stainless steel water bottle. But, be careful. Many products on the market are lined with an epoxy finish. This defeats the purpose. Make sure that the bottle is stainless steel both inside and out. Stainless steel water bottles are light, durable, and hold both hot and cold liquids well. My favorite stainless steel water bottle can be found at www.holisticphysician.com/onlinestore/waterfilters/new_ wave_enviro/polycarbonate_plastic_containers.htm.

The second approach is to reuse glass containers such as quart-sized juice bottles. Yes, they are a bit heavier but are good solutions if you're in an office environment where mobility isn't an issue. Or you can buy glass water bottles. Check out the following link to Aquasana AQ6000 Glass Water Bottles: www.medmarketplace.com/aquasana-aq6000-glass-water-bottles-set-of-six-29709.html.

Recommended Reading

Books

If you have not already done so, I strongly recommend that you read my first book, *From Hormone Hell to Hormone Well*. In it I provide you with an even stronger foundation regarding the safety and efficacy of bio-identical hormone replacement. You may purchase it on line via my website, www.hormonewell.com, through www.amazon.com, or at your local bookstore.

In addition, there are many other physician pioneers and medical experts who have helped lay a foundation of learning and knowledge regarding bio-identical hormone therapy. I have the following books in my personal library. Each author offers the reader the benefit of additional information and another perspective. Please note that these resources are not prioritized by perceived merit but are listed in alphabetical order according to author.

Lee, John R., M.D., *Natural Progesterone, The Multiple Role of a Remarkable Hormone.* Sebastopol, CA: BLL Publishing, 1993.

Lee, John R., M.D., with Jesse Hanley, M.D., and Virginia Hopkins. *What Your Doctor May Not Tell You About Perimenopause.* New York: Warner Books, 1999.

Lee, John R., M.D., with Virginia Hopkins. *What Your Doctor May Not Tell You About Menopause.* New York: Warner Books, 1996.

Lee, John R., M.D., with David Zava, Ph.D., and Virginia Hopkins. *What Your Doctor May Not Tell You About Breast Cancer.* New York: Warner Books, 2002.

Northrup, Christiane, M.D., *The Wisdom of Menopause: Creating Physical and Emotional Health and Healing During the Change.* New York: Bantam Books, 2001.

Northrup, Christiane, M.D., *Women's Bodies, Women's Wisdom: Creating Physical and Emotional Health and Healing.* New York: Bantam Books, 1994.

Schwartz, Erika, M.D., *The Hormone Solution.* New York: Warner Books, 2002.

Seaman, Barbara. *The Greatest Experiment Ever Performed on Women: Exploding the Estrogen Myth.* New York: Hyperion Books, 2003.

Shulman, Neil, M.D., and Kim S. Edmunds, M.D., *Healthy Transitions: A Woman's Guide to Perimenopause, Menopause & Beyond.* New York: Prometheus Books, 2004.

Somers, Suzanne, *The Sexy Years, Discover the Hormone Connection: The Secret to Fabulous Sex, Great Health, and Vitality for Women and Men.* New York: Crown Publishers, 2004.

Taylor, Eldred, M.D., and Ava Bell-Taylor, M.D., *Are Your Hormone Making You Sick?* Physicians Natural Medicine, Inc., 2000.

Whitaker, Julian, M.D., *Dr. Whitaker's Guide to Natural Hormone Replacement.* Potomac, MD: Phillips Publishing, 1999.

Wilson, James L., N.D., D.C., Ph.D., *Adrenal Fatigue.* Petaluma, CA: Smart Publications, 2003.

Wright, Jonathan V., M.D., and John Morgenthaler, *Natural Hormone Replacement for Women Over 45.* Petaluma, CA: Smart Publications, 1997.

Newsletters

E-mail newsletters can be a great source of new information regarding hormone health. They can also serve as excellent reminders of good information you might have read once but have forgotten. There are several excellent newsletters available today. I recommend that you check out and sign up for:

My own. You can register to receive my free monthly newsletter via my website: www.hormonewell.com

Women in Balance: www.womeninbalance.org

Virginia Hopkin's Healthwatch: www.virginiahopkins healthwatch.com

The Natural Progesterone Advisory Network: www. natural-progesterone-advisory-network.com

Best Resource: Yourself

In closing, I want to take a minute to remind each reader that no one can tell you what is right for you, your body, or for your health. I encourage you to read, ask questions, and do your homework. While it is my privilege to be your resource, when it comes to your health and well-being only *you* can be your own final authority.

REFERENCES

Abdulla, M., and P. Gruber. "Role of Diet Modification in Cancer Prevention." *Biofactors* 12 (2000): 45–51.

Abraham, G. E., and R. E. Rumley. "The Role of Nutrition in Managing the Premenstrual Tension Syndromes." *Journal of Reproductive Medicine* 32 (1987): 405–22.

Alam, I., K. Lewis, J. W. Stephens, and J. N. Baxter. "Obesity, Metabolic Syndrome and Sleep Apnoea: All Pro-inflammatory States." *Obesity Review* 8, no. 2 (2007): 119–27.

Allison, D. B., G. Gadbury, L. G. Schwartz, R. Murugesan, J. L. Kraker, S. Heshka, K. R. Fontaine, and S. B. Heymsfield. "A Novel Soy-Based Meal Replacement Formula for Weight Loss Among Obese Individuals: A Randomized Controlled Clinical Trial." *European Journal of Clinical Nutrition* 57 (2003): 514–22.

Angell, M. *The Truth About the Drug Companies*. New York: Random House, 2005.

Ann, N. Y. *Mind-Body Medicine: Stress and Its Impact on Overall Health and Longevitiy*. New York: New York Academy of Sciences, 2005.

Appleby, M. "Why Drinking Water Is Really the Key to Weight Loss." www.inch-aweigh.com, 2006.

Aronson, D. "Take the Right Vitamins for You." *Natural Health* (August 2003): 67–77.

Babal, K. "Reversing Liver Damage: The Body's Largest Detox Organ Needs Repair Work Now and Then." *Nutrition Science News* (October 1997).

Balch, J., and P. Balch. *Prescription for Nutritional Healing: A-to-Z Guide to Supplements*. Garden City Park, NY: Avery, 1998.

Barbosa, J. C., T. D. Shultz, S. J. Filley, and D. C. Neiman. "The Relationship Among Adiposity, Diet, and Hormone Concentrations in Vegetarian and Nonvegetarian Postmenopausal Women." *American Journal of Clinical Nutrition* 51 (1990): 798–803.

Barrett-Connor, E., and T. L. Bush. "Estrogen and Coronary Heart Disease in Women." *Journal of the American Medical Association* 265 (1991): 1861–67.

Barrett-Connor, E., D. Grady, and M. L. Sefanik. "The Rise and Fall of Menopausal Hormone Therapy." *Annual Review of Public Health* 26 (2005): 115–40.

Batterham, Rachel. *Journal of Cell Metabolism* (2006).

Benson, H., and E. M. Stuart. *The Wellness Book*. New York: Fireside, 1992.

Biskin, M. S. "Nutritional Deficiency in the Etiology of Menorrhagia, Metrorrhagia, Cystic Mastitis and Premenstrual Tension: Treatment with Vitamin B Complex." *Journal of Clinical Endocrinology Metabolism* 3 (1943): 227.

Blair, S., H. Kohl, R. Paffenbarger, D. Clark, K. Cooper, and L. Gibbons.

"Physical Fitness and All-Cause Mortality: A Prospective Study of Healthy Men and Women." *Journal of the American Medical Association* 262 (1989): 2395–2401.

Blumenthal, J., R. Williams, T. Needles, and A. Wallace. "Psychological Changes Acompanying Aerobic Exercise in Healthy Middle-Aged Adults." *Psychosomatic Medicine* 44 (1982): 529–36.

Boggiano, M. M., A. I. Artiga, C. E. Pritchett, P. C. Chandler-Laney, M. L. Smith, and A. J. Eldridge. "High Intake of Palatable Food Predicts Binge-Eating Independent of Susceptibility to Obesity: An Animal Model of Lean vs. Obese Binge-Eating and Obesity With and Without Binge-Eating." *International Journal of Obesity.* (2007).

Borysenko, J. *Minding the Body, Mending the Mind.* Reading, MA: Addison-Wesley, 1987.

Campana, W. M., and C. R. Baumrucker. *Handbook of Milk Composition: Hormones and Growth Factors in Bovine Milk.* New York: Academic Press, 1995.

Chang, M. I. W. "Dietary Pectic: Effect on Metabolic Processes in Rats." In *Unconventional Sources of Dietary Fiber,* edited by I. Furda. Washington, DC: American Chemical Society, 1983.

Chen, I., S. Safe, and L. Bjeldanes. "Indole-3-Carbinol and Diindolylmethane as Aryl Hydrocarbon Receptor Agonists and Antagonists in T47D Human Breast Cancer Cells." *Journal of the National Cancer Institute* 7 (1996): 1069–76.

Cho, E. J., Y. A. Lee, H. H. Yoo, and T. Yokozawa. "Protective Effects of Broccoli Against Oxidative Damage in Vitro and in Vivo." *Journal of Nutritional Scientific Vitaminology* 52, no. 6 (2006): 437–44.

Colbert, D. *The Bible Cure for Thyroid Disorders.* Lake Mary, FL: Siloam, 2004.

Collins, K. "How Whole Grains Can Fight Disease." Available online at www.msnbc.msn.com/id/7080356.

Deibert , P., D. Konig, A. Schmidt-Trucksaess, K. S. Zaenker, I. Frey, U. Landmann, and A. Berg. "Weight Loss Without Losing Muscle Mass in Pre-obese and Obese Subjects Induced by a High-Soy-Protein Diet." *International Journal of Obesity* 28 (2004): 1349–52.

Diamond, J. *Surviving Male Menopause.* Naperville, IL: Sourcebooks, 2000.

Dossey, L. *Reinventing Medicine: Beyond Mind-Body to a New Era of Healing.* San Francisco: HarperSanFrancisco, 1999.

Dubey, R. K., D. G. Gillespie, E. K. Jackson, and Paul J. Keller. "17B-Estradiol, Its Metabolites, and Progesterone Inhibit Cardiac Fibroblast Growth." *Hypertension* 31 (1998): 522. Available online at www.ahajournals.org.

Edwards, C. "Mechanisms of Action on Dietary Fiber on Small Intestinal Absorption and Motility." In *New Development in Dietary Fiber.* New York: Plenum Press, 1990.

Eisenstein, J., S. B. Roberts, G. Dallal, and E. Saltzman. "Structured Weight-Loss Programs: Meta-Analysis of Weight Loss at 24 Weeks and Assessment of Effects of Intervention Intensity." *Advanced Therapy* 21 (2004): 61–75.

Elkins, R. *Nature's Phen-Fen: Natural Supplements for Losing Weight.* Pleasant Grove, UT: Woodland Publishing, 1997.

Epstein, S. "American Beef: Why Is It Banned in Europe?" Available online at http://preventcancer.com/consumers/general/hormones_meat.htm.

Fontaine, K. R., D. Yang, G. L. Gadbury, S. Heshka, L. G. Schwartz, R. Murugesan, J. L. Kraker, M. Heo, S. B. Heymsfield, and D. B. Allison. "Results of a Soy-Based Meal Replacement Formula on Weight, Anthropometry, Serum Lipids and Blood Pressure During a 40-week Clinical Weight-Loss Trial." *European Journal of Clinical Nutrition* 57 (2003): 514–22.

Fournier, L. R., R. Borchers, L. M. Robison, M. Wiediger, J. S. Park, B. P. Chew, M. K. McGuire, D. A. Sclar, T. L. Skaer, and K. A. Beerman. "The Effects of Soy Milk and Isoflavone Supplements on Cognitive Performance in Healthy, Postmenopausal Women." *Journal of Nutrition, Health, and Aging* 11, no. 2 (2007): 155–64.

Friel, P. N., C. Hinchcliffe, and J. V. Wright. "Hormone Replacement with Estradiol: Conventional Oral Doses Result in Excessive Exposure to Estrogen." *Alternative Medical Review* 10 (2005): 36–41.

Fukada,Y., K. Kimura, and Y. Ayaki. "Effects of chitosan feeding on intestinal bile acid metabolism in rats." *Lipids* 20 (1991): 395–99.

Furda, I. "Interaction of Dietary Fiber with Lipids: Mechanic Theories and Their Limitations." In *New Developments in Dietary Fiber.* New York: Plenum Press, 1990.

Gandhi, R., and S. M. Snedeker. "Consumer Concerns About Hormones in Food." Available online at http://envirocancer.cornell.edu/Factsheet/Diet/fs37.hormones.cfm.

Garry, P. J., R. N. Baumgartner, S. G. Brodie, G. D. Montoya, H. C. Liang, R. D. Lindeman, and T. M. Williams. "Estrogen Replacement Therapy, Serum Lipids, and Polymorphism of the Apolipoprotein E Gene." *Clinical Chemistry* 45 (1999): 1214–23. Available online at www.Clinichem.org.

Gaudet, T. W., P. Spencer, and A. Weil. *Consciously Female.* New York: Bantam Books, 2004.

Gearon, C. J. "Midlife or Menopause?" Available online at http://health.discovery.com/centers/mens/articles/andropause.html.

Geim, C., U. Ehlert, and D. H. Hellhammer. "The Potential Role of Hypocortisolism in the Pathophysiology of Stress-Related Bodily Disorders." *Psychoneuroendocrinology* 25, no. 1 (2000): 1–35.

Giuca, L. "Nothing Complex About Choosing the Right Carbohydrates in Diet." *The Milwaukee Journal Sentinel,* 1999. Available online at www.findarticles.com/p/articles/mi_qn4196/is_19990117/ai_n10494852.

Goldin, B. R., H. Adlercreutz, J. T. Dwyer, L. Swenson, J. H. Warram, and S. L. Gorbach. "Effect of Diet on Excretion of Estrogens in Peri- and Postmenopausal Women." *Cancer Research* 14 (1981): 3771–73.

Goldin, B. R., and S. L. Gorbach. "Effect of Diet on the Plasma Levels, Metabolism, and Excretion of Estrogens." *American Journal of Clinical Nutrition* 48 (1988): 787–90.

Goldstein, J., C. K. Sites, and M. J. Toth. "Progesterone Stimulates Cardiac Muscle Protein Synthesis via Receptor-Dependent Pathway." *Fertility and Sterility* 82, no. 2 (2004): 430–36. Available online at www.sciencedirect.com.

Graham, J. "How Stress Makes You Fat." *Ladies Home Journal* (July 2005): 168–74.

Greider, K. *The Big Fix.* New York: Public Affairs, 2003.

Grossman, T. *The Baby Boomers' Guide to Living Forever.* Golden, CO: Hubristic Press, 2000.

Hawthorne, F. *Inside the FDA.* Hoboken, NJ: John Wiley & Sons, 2005.

Holm R. R., and P. Bjorntorp. "Food-Induced Cortisol Secretion in Relation to Anthropometric, Metabolic and Haemodynamic Variables in Men." *International Journal of Obesity-Related Metabolic Disorders* 24, no. 4 (2000): 416–22.

Holmes, M. "Adrenal Fatigue: The Effects of Stress and High Cortisol Levels." *Women to Women* (2006): 1–4.

Hoy, C. *The Truth About Breast Cancer.* Ontario, Canada: Stoddart, 1996.

Igimi, H., M. Nishimura, R. Kodama, and H. Ide. "Studies on the Metabolism of d-Limonene: The Absorption, Distribution, and Exvertion of d-Limonene in Rats." *Xenobiotica* 4, no. 2 (1974): 77–84.

Ikeda, I., M. Sugano, K. Yoshida, E. Sasaki, Y. Iwamoto, and K. Hatano. "Effects of Chitosan Hydrolysates on Lipid Absorption and on Serum and Liver Lipid Concentrations in Rats." *Journal of Agricultural and Food Chemistry* 41 (1993): 431–435.

Ingram, D. M., F. C. Bennett, D. Wilcox, and N. de Klerk. "Effect of Low-Fat Diet on Female Sex Hormone Levels." *Journal of the National Cancer Institute* 79 (1987): 1225–29.

Jenness, R. "Composition of Milk." In *Fundamentals of Dairy Chemistry*, edited by N. P. Wong, R. Jenness, J. Kenney, and E. H. Marth. New York: Reinhold, 1988.

Jeong, H. J., Y. G. Shin, I. H. Kim, and J. M. Pezzuto. "Inhibition of Aromatase Activity by Flavonoids." *Archives of Pharmacological Research* 22 (1999): 309–12.

Kannel, W. B., M. C. Hjortland, P. M. McNamara, and T. Gordon. "Menopause and Risk of Cardiovascular Disease: The Framingham Study." *Annals of International Medicine* 85 (1976): 447–452.

Kao, Y. C., C. Zhou, M. Sherman, C. A. Laughton, and S. Chen. "Molecular Basis of the Inhibition of Human Aromatase by Flavone and Isoflavone Phytoestrogens: A Site-Directed Mutagenesis Study." *Environmental Health Perspectives* 106, no. 2 (1998): 85–92.

Kellis, J. T., and L. E. Vickery. "Inhibition of Human Estrogen Synthetase by Flavones." *Science* 225, no. 4666 (1984): 1032–34.

Kelly, J., D. Kaufman, K. Kelly, L. Rosenberg, T. Anderson, and A. Mitchell. "Recent Trends in Use of Herbal and Other Natural Products." *Archives of Internal Medicine* 165, no. 3 (2005). Available online at http://archinte.amaassa.org/cgi/content/abstract/165/3/281.

Keys, A., and M. Keys. *How to Eat Well and Stay Well the Mediterranean Way.* Garden City, NY: Doubleday, 1975.

Knorr, D. "Recovery and Utilization of Chitin and Chitosan in Food Processing Waste Management." *Food Technology* 45 (1991): 114–22.

Kodama, R., A. Okubo, E. Araki, K. Noda, H. Ide, and T. Ikeda. "Studies on the Metabolism of d-Limonene as a Gallstone Solubilizer: Effects on

Development of Mouse Fetuses and Offspring." *Oyo Yakuri* 13, no. 6 (1977): 863–73.

Lee, J. R. *Natural Progesterone: The Multiple Role of a Remarkable Hormone.* Sebastopol, CA: BLL Publishing, 1993.

Lee, J. R., J. Hanley, and V. Hopkins. *What Your Doctor May Not Tell You About Perimenopause: Balance Your Hormones and Your Life from Thirty to Fifty.* New York: Warner Books, 1999.

Lee, J. R., and V. Hopkins. *What Your Doctor May Not Tell You About Menopause.* New York: Warner Books, 1996.

Lee, J. R., D. Zava, and V. Hopkins. *What Your Doctor May Not Tell You About Breast Cancer: How Hormone Balance Can Help Save Your Life.* New York: Warner Books, 2002.

Leon, A., J. Connett, D. Jacobs, and R. Rauramaa. "Leisure-Time Physical Activity Levels and Risk of Coronary Heart Disease and Death: The Multiple Risk Factor Intervention Trial." *Journal of the American Medical Association* 258 (1987): 2388–95.

Leonetti, H. B., S. Longo, and J. N. Anasti. "Transdermal Progesterone Cream for Vasomotor Symptoms and Postmenopausal Bone Loss." *Obstretrics and Gynecology* 94 (1999): 225–28.

Lerner, M. *Choices in Healing: Integrating the Best of Conventional and Complementary Approaches to Cancer.* Cambridge, MA: MIT Press, 1994.

Lewis, T. T., S. A. Everson-Rose, B. Sternfeld, K. Karavolos, D. Wesley, and L. H. Powell. "Race, Education, and Weight Change in a Briacia Sample of Women at Midlife." *Archives of Internal Medicine* 165 (2005): 545–51.

Lopez, D., M. D. Sanchez, W. Shea-Eaton, and M. P. McLean. "Estrogen Activates the High Density Lipoprotein Receptor Gene via Binding to Estrogen Response Elements and Interaction with Sterol Regulatory Element Binding Protein-1A." *Endocrinology* 143 (2002): 2155–68.

Maezaki, Y., K. Tusuji, Y. Nakagawa, Y. Kawai, and M. Akimoto. "Hypocholesterolemic Effect of Chitosan in Adult Males." *Bioscience, Biotechnology and Biochemistry* 57 (1993): 1439–44.

Manson, J. E, and S. Bassuk. *Hot Flashes, Hormones & Your Health.* New York: McGraw-Hill, 2007.

McKwoen, N. M., J. B. Meigs, S. Liu, E. Saltzman, P. W. Wilson, and P. F. Jacques. "Carbohydrate Nutrition, Insulin Resistance, and the Prevalence of the Metabolic Syndrome in the Framingham Offspring Cohort." *Diabetes Care* 27 (2004): 518–46.

Mendelsohn, M. E., and R. H. Karas. "The Protective Effects of Estrogen on the Cardiovascular System." *New England Journal of Medicine* 340 (1999): 1801–11.

Miller, V. M., D. J. Tindall, and P. Y. Liu. "Of Mice, Men, and Hormones." *Arteriosclerosis, Thrombosis, and Vascular Biology* 24 (2004): 995.

Morales, A. J., R. H. Hubrich, and J. Y. Hwang. "The Effect of Six Months' Treatment with a 100 mg Daily Dose of Dehydroepiandrosterone on Circulating Sex Steroids." *Clinical Endocrinology* 29 (1998): 421–32.

Morales, A. J., J. J. Nolan, J. C. Nelson, and S. S. C. Yen. "Effects of Replacement Dose of DHEA in Men and Women of Advancing Age." *Journal of Clinical Endocrinology Metabolism* 78 (1994): 1360.

Myers, H. F, T. T. Lewis, and T. Parker-Dominguez. *Stress, Coping and Minority Health: Biopsychosocial Perspectives on Ethnic Health Disparities.*

Thousand Oaks, CA: Sage Publications, 2003.

Nestler, J. E., C. O. Barlascini, J. N. Clore, and W. G. Blackard. "Dehydroepiandrosterone Reduces Serum Low Density Lipoprotein Levels and Body Fat but Does Not Alter Insulin Sensitivity in Normal Men." *Journal of Clinical Endocrinology Metabolism* 66 (1988): 57–61.

Nhat, H. T., *Being Peace*. Berkeley, CA: Parallaz Press, 1987.

Northrup, C. *The Wisdom of Menopause: Creating Physical and Emotional Health and Healing During the Change*. New York: Bantam, 2001.

Northrup, C. *Women's Bodies, Women's Wisdom: Creating Physical and Emotional Health and Healing*. New York: Bantam Books, 1994.

Opdyke, D. J. L. "Monographs on Fragrance Raw Materials." *Food and Cosmetics* 13 (1975): 825–26.

Park, S. J., L. T. Goldsmith, J. H. Skurnick, G. Weiss, and A. Wojtczuk. "Characteristics of the Urinary Luteinizing Hormone Surge in Young Ovulatory Women." *Fertility and Sterility* (2007).

Pathak, N., S. Khandelwal. "Role of Oxidative Stress and Apoptosis in Cadmium Induced Thymic Atrophy and Splenomegaly in Mice." *Toxicology* 169, no. 2 (2007): 95–108.

Pelissero, C., M. J. Lenczowski, D. Chinzi, B. Davail-Cuisset, and J. P. Sumpter. "Fostier Effects of Flavonoids on Aromatase Activity: An in Vitro Study." *Journal of Steroidal, Biochemical, and Molecular Biology* 57 (1996): 215–23.

Plechner, A. J. "Cortisol Abnormality as a Cause of Elevated Estrogen and Immune Destabilization: Insights for Human Medicine from a Veterinary Perspective." *Medical Hypotheses* 62, no. 4 (2004): 575–81.

Prentice, R., F. C. Bennett, C. Clifford, S. Gorbach, B. Goldin, and D. Byar. "Dietary Fat Reduction and Plasma Estradiol Concentration in Healthy Postmenopausal Women." *Journal of the National Cancer Institute* 82 (1990). 129–34.

Purohit, A., H. A. Hejaz, and L. Walden. "The Effect of 2-Methoxyoestrone-3-O-Sulphamate on the Growth of Breast Cancer Cells and Induced Mammary Tumours." *International Journal of Cancer* 85 (2000): 584–89.

Raloff, J. "Hormones in Your Milk." *Science News Online* 164, no. 18 (2003). Available online at http://sciencenews.org/articles/20031101/food.asp.

Randall, M. "Hormones and Belly Fat." Available online at http://abc.net.au/overnights/stories/s1258936.htm.

Randolph, Jr., C.W., and G. James. *From Hormone Hell to Hormone Well*. Jacksonville Beach, FL: Natural Hormone Institute of America, 2004.

Ray, A., R. Semba, J. Walston, L. Ferrucci, A. Cappola, M. Ricks, Q. L. Xue, and L. Fried. "Low Serum Selenium and Total Carotenoids Predict Mortality Among Older Women Living in the Community: The Women's Health and Aging Studies." *American Society for Nutrition* 136 (2006): 172–76. Available online at http://jn.nutrition.org/cgi/content/abstract/136/1/172.

Razdan, A., and D. Pattersson. "Effect of Chitin and Chitosan on Nutrient Digestibility and Plasma Lipid Concentrations in Broiler Chickens." *British Journal of Nutrition* 72 (1994): 277–88.

Reiss, U., and M. Zucker. *Natural Hormone Balance for Women*. New York: Pocket Books, 2001.

references

Remer, T., and F. Manz. "Estimation of the Renal Net Acid Excretion by Adults Consuming Diets Containing Variable Amounts of Protein." *Amerian Journal of Clinical Nutrition* 59 (1994): 1356–61.

Renland, J. G., and P. E. Johnson. "Dietary Calcium and Manganese Effects on Menstrual Cycle Symptoms." *American Journal of Obstetrics and Gynecology* 168 (1993): 141.

Rose, D. P., J. R. Loughridge, C. Cohen, and L. E. Strong. "Effect of Low-Fat Diet on Female Sex Hormone Levels in Women with Cystic Breast Disease." *Journal of the National Cancer Institute* 78 (1987): 623–26.

Rowen, R. "Redesigned Supplement Fights Breast and Prostate Cancer." *Dr. Robert Jay Rowen's Second Opinion* 15, no. 8 (2005).

Sahelian, R. "New Supplements and Unknown, Long-Term Consequences." *American Journal of Natural Medicine* 4 (1997): 8.

Saunders, Dave. "A View of the Mediterranean Diet Pyramid." Available online at www.changingshape.com/resources/articles/the-mediterranean-diet.asp.

Schoppen, B., A. Carbajal, A. Perez-Granados, F. Vivas, and M. Vaquero. "Food, Energy and Macronutrient Intake of Postmenopausal Women from a Menopause Program." *Nutricion Hospitalaria* 20, no. 2 (2005): 101–109.

Schulze, M. B., S. Liu, E. B. Rimm, J. E. Manson, W. C. Willett, and F. B. Hu. "Glycemic Index, Glycemic Load, and Dietary Fiber Intake and Incidence of Type 2 Diabetes in Younger and Middle-Aged Women." *American Journal of Clinical Nutrition* 80 (2004): 348–56.

Schwartz, E. *The Hormone Solution.* New York: Warner Books, 2002.

Seaman, B. *The Greatest Experiment Ever Performed on Women: Exploding the Estrogen Myth.* New York: Hyperion Books, 2003.

Shomon, M. "Do Soy Foods Negatively Affect Your Thyroid?" Available online at http://thyroid-info.com/articles/soydangers.htm.

Shulman, N., and K. S. Edmunds. *Healthy Transitions: A Woman's Guide to Perimenopause, Menopause & Beyond.* New York: Prometheus Books, 2004.

Shultz, T. D., and J. E. Leklem. "Nutrient Intake and Hormonal Status of Premenopausal Vegetarian Seventh-Day Adventists and Premenopausal Nonvegetarians." *Nutrition and Cancer* 4 (1983): 247–59.

Somers, S. *The Sexy Years, Discover the Hormone Connection: The Secret to Fabulous Sex, Great Health, and Vitality for Women and Men.* New York: Crown Publishers, 2004.

Sun, Y., C. Gu, X. Lui, W. Liang, P. Yao, J. L. Bolton, and R. B. van Breemen. "Ultrafiltration Tandem Mass Spectrometry of Estrogens for Characterization of Structure and Affinity for Human Estrogen Receptors." *PubMed Central* 16, no. 2 (2005): 271–79. Available online at www.Pubmedcentral.nih.gov.

Taylor, E. B., and A. Bell-Taylor. *Are Your Hormones Making You Sick?* Physicians' Natural Medicine, 2000.

Teta, J., and K. Teta. "The Impact of Lifestyle Choices and Hormonal Balance on Coping with Stress." *The Townsend Letter* (2005).

Trichopoulou, A., T. Costacou, C. Bamia, and D. Trichopoulou. "Adherence to a Mediterranean Diet and Survival in a Greek Population." *The New England Journal of Medicine* 348, no. 26 (2003): 2599-2608.

Tsuji, M., Y. Fujisaki, and Y. Arikawa. "Studies on the Metabolism of d-Limonene as a Gallstone Solubilizer: Chronic Toxicity in Rats." *Oyo Yakuri* 9, no. 3 (1975): 403–412.

Uebelhack, R., J. U. Blohmer, H. J. Graubaum, R. Busch, J. Gruenwald, and K. D. Wernecke. "Black Cohosh and St. John's Wort for Climacteric Complaints." *Obstetrics and Gynecology* 107 (2006): 247–55.

Usiskin, K. S., S. Butterworth, and J. N. Clore. "Lack of Effect of Dehydroepiandrosterone in Obese Men." *International Journal of Obesity* 14 (1990): 457–63.

Vaillant, G. E. *Aging Well.* Boston: Little, Brown, 2002.

Van Duyn, M. A., and E. Pivonka. "Overview of the Health Benefits of Fruit and Vegetable Consumption for the Dietetics Professional: Selected Literature." *Journal of the American Dietary Association* 100 (2000): 1511–21.

Weil, A. *Eating Well for Optimum Health: The Essential Guide to Bringing Health and Pleasure Back to Eating.* New York: Quill, 2001.

Whitaker, J. *Dr. Whitaker's Guide to Natural Hormone Replacement.* Potomac, MD: Phillips Publishing, 1999.

Wilson, J. L. *Adrenal Fatigue.* Petaluma, CA: Smart Publications, 2001.

Wren, B. G., K. McFarland, and L. Edwards. "Micronised Transdermal Progesterone and Endometria Response." *Lancet* 354 (1999): 1447–48.

Wright, J. V., and J. Morgenthaler. *Natural Hormone Replacement for Women Over 45.* Petaluma, CA: Smart Publications, 1997.

Zimecki, M., and M. L. Kruzel. "Milk-Derived Proteins and Peptides of Potential Therapeutic and Nutritive Value." *Journal of Experimental Therapeutics and Oncology* 6, no. 2 (2007): 86–106.

INDEX

Page numbers followed by an *f* or a *t* indicate figures or tables.

abdominal fat. *See* belly fat
absorption
    calcium D-glucarate and, 89–90
    calcium-magnesium combo,
        92–93
    water and, 36
acetaldehyde, 198
acetone, 198
Activella, 75
estrogen dominance and, 18
activity, physical. *See* physical activity
Adrenal Boost, 112–13
adrenal function
    bio-identical hormone
        replacement and, 75
    progesterone and, 9
    steroids and, 7
    stress and, 103
    support of, 112–13
aerobics, 112
age
    bio-identical hormone
        replacement therapies and, 115
    dehydroepiandrosterone and,
        93–94
    estrogen dominance and, 4, 9,
        12–14, 17
    premature aging and, 15
air filters, 199
air fresheners, 198
alcohol, 39, 40, 198
aldehydes, 198
aliphatic hydrocarbons, 198
almonds
    as part of diet plan, 44, 48, 50,
        54, 59, 65, 69, 71
    as protein source, 32*t*

as source of calcium, 35*t*
Alzheimer's disease, synthetic
    hormone replacement and, 76
American Cancer Society, 80
American Liver Association, 39
andropause, 13
Angell, Marcia, 77
anovulation, 17
antidepressants
    estrogen dominance and, 19–20
    need for, 4
    progesterone as, 6
antioxidants, fruits and, 35
anxiety
    antidepressants and, 20
    bio-identical progesterone and,
        83
    cortisol and, 111
    estrogen dominance and, 14
    hormone balance and, 15
Appleby, Maia, 37
apples
    Cabbage-Apple Salad, 173
    as important food to reduce
        estrogen dominance, 27, 35
    as part of diet plan, 43, 45, 47,
        48, 51, 55, 56, 58, 60, 63, 64,
        65, 66, 69, 72
    Turkey, Apple, and Spinach
        Pita, 149
Aquasana, 215
Arbonne International, 204
aromatic hydrocarbons, 198
arugula, as important food to
    reduce estrogen dominance,
    29–30*t*
Asian Cabbage, 151

asparagus
  Asparagus Omelet, 122
  Chicken and Asparagus
    Lettuce Wraps, 127
  Dressed-Up Asparagus, 157
  Grilled Asparagus with Sesame
    Seeds, 160
  as important food to reduce
    estrogen dominance, 26,
    29–30t
  as part of diet plan, 43, 46, 47,
    48, 50, 53, 59, 60, 61, 63, 64,
    67, 70
  Skillet Broccoli or Asparagus
    with Sesame Seeds, 169
  Turkey and Asparagus Wraps,
    148
Asparagus Omelet, 122
avocados
  Grapefruit and Avocado Salad,
    182
  as important food to reduce
    estrogen dominance, 35
  as part of diet plan, 44
Avon, 213
Ayurvedic medicine, water and,
  36–37

B vitamins, 90–91, 112
bacon
  Cauliflower and Turkey Bacon
    Soup, 125
  Pan-Roasted Fish with Parsley
    and Turkey Bacon, 141
  as part of diet plan, 46, 48, 50,
    53, 60, 61, 67, 69, 71
  Tossed Turkey Bacon and
    Spinach Salad, 146
bacteria
  lignans and, 28
  soluble fiber and, 27
Baked Fish with Basil, 123
Baked Rutabaga, 152
Banana in Bark, 171
bananas
  as important food to reduce
    estrogen dominance, 35
  as part of diet plan, 46, 52, 55,
    59, 67

barley, as important food to
    reduce estrogen dominance,
    27, 29–30t
Batterham, Rachel, 31
BCL2, 79
beans. See also specific varieties
  Best Baked Beans, 154
  Black Beanofritos, 124
  as important food to reduce
    estrogen dominance, 27
  Nest of Beans and Greens, 137
  as part of diet plan, 45, 50, 57,
    61, 65, 66, 71
  as protein source, 32, 32t
  as source of calcium, 35t
  Spicy Kale and Beans, 145
beef
  as part of diet plan, 46, 53, 67
  as protein source, 31–32, 32t
Beet and Orange Salad, 172
beet root
  Beet and Orange Salad, 172
  Beets and Brussels Sprouts, 153
  Easy Pickled Beets, 158
  Grated Beet Salad, 183
  as important food to reduce
    estrogen dominance, 26,
    29–30t
  as part of diet plan, 43, 49, 52,
    55, 58, 65, 67, 70
  Roasted Beets, 166
  Spinach Salad with Beets in
    Cottage Cheese, 188
Beets and Brussels Sprouts, 153
  belching, water and, 36
belly fat
  estrogen dominance and (see
    estrogen dominance)
  hormone balance and, 15
benzene, 198
berries
  as important food to reduce
    estrogen dominance, 27, 35
  as part of diet plan, 42, 44, 49,
    54, 57, 58, 60, 61, 62, 65, 70
Best Baked Beans, 154
beverages. See alcohol; caffeine;
    juices; water

Beverly Hills Anti-Aging Center, 79
BHRT. *See* bio-identical hormone
    replacement therapies
bi-est, 119–20
biking, 112
bio-identical hormone
    replacement therapies
    80-20 rule of, 115–20
    as alternative to synthetic,
        74–76
    hormone replacement and, 19
    patenting and, 20–21
    progesterone and (*see*
        progesterone)
    recent attention regarding, 74
birth control pills
    avoiding use of, 199
    as hormone replacement, 19
    as toxin, 16
    xenoestrogen and, 18
bisphenol-A, 214
Black Beanofritos, 124
black beans
    Black Beanofritos, 124
    as part of diet plan, 52, 60
    as protein source, 32*t*
black-eyed peas
    as protein source, 32*t*
    as source of calcium, 35*t*
bloating
    antidepressants and, 20
    estrogen dominance and, 13, 17
    progesterone and, 6
    water and, 36
blood clotting, calcium-
        magnesium combo and,
        92–93
blood sugar, 31
blueberries, as important food to
        reduce estrogen dominance,
        27, 35
The Body Shop, 213
bok choy, as important food to
        reduce estrogen dominance,
        29–30*t*
bone health, progesterone and, 6
bottles, 214–15
BPA. *See* bisphenol-A

Brazil nuts, as protein source, 32*t*
bread
    as important food to reduce
        estrogen dominance, 27
    as part of diet plan, 42, 43, 44,
        47, 50, 51, 53, 55, 59, 63, 64,
        65, 68, 71, 72
breakfast. *See* monthly diet plan
breast cancer
    progesterone and, 6
    The Truth About Breast Cancer
        and, 22
breast tenderness
    estrogen dominance and, 14
    hormone balance and, 15
    vitamin E and, 91–92
breathing, stress and, 107–8
Breus, Michael, 111
broccoli
    Broccoli and Cauliflower in
        Lime Dressing, 155
    as important food to reduce
        estrogen dominance, 26,
        29–30*t*
    Marinated Broccoli, Cucumber,
        and Tomato Salad, 164
    as part of diet plan, 43, 44, 46,
        48, 53, 60, 62, 64, 71
    Skillet Broccoli or Asparagus
        with Sesame Seeds, 169
Broccoli and Cauliflower in Lime
    Dressing, 155
brown rice
    Chicken and Cold Rice Salad, 175
    as important food to reduce
        estrogen dominance, 27,
        29–30*t*
    as part of diet plan, 42, 47, 57,
        58, 60, 63, 66, 68, 70
    Spinach and Feta Brown Rice, 170
Brussels sprouts
    Beets and Brussels Sprouts, 153
    as important food to reduce
        estrogen dominance, 26,
        29–30*t*
    Indian-Style Brussels Sprouts,
        161
    as part of diet plan, 45, 51, 58, 72

buffalo, as part of diet plan, 53
burn out, hormone balance and,
    15
butter, avoiding, 36

cabbage
    Asian Cabbage, 151
    Cabbage-Apple Salad, 173
    Creamy Coleslaw, 177
    as important food to reduce
        estrogen dominance, 26,
        29–30t
    Kale and Sauerkraut, 162
    as part of diet plan, 45, 49, 51,
        52, 56, 57, 58, 64, 66, 68, 72
    Quick Turkey-Stuffed Cabbage,
        142
    Sauerkraut Salad, 186
Cabbage-Apple Salad, 173
caffeine, 38–39, 40
    supplements and, 92–93
calcium
    calcium D-glucarate, 89–90
    calcium-magnesium combo,
        92–93
    as important to reducing
        estrogen dominance, 33–35,
        37
    sources of, 35t
calming agent, progesterone as, 6
Campaign for Safe Cosmetics, 212
cancer
    bio-identical progesterone and,
        78–79
    calcium D-glucarate and, 89–90
    estrogen and, 21–22
    estrone and, 76
    progesterone and, 6
Cancer Detection and Prevention
    Journal, 76
canola oil, calcium-magnesium
    combo and, 92–93
capillary blood spot testing, 206
capsules, bio-identical
    progesterone and, 83. See
    also progesterone
car exhausts, xenoestrogen and, 16
carbohydrates

blood sugar and, 31
    estrogen and, 38
carbon tetrachloride, 198
cardiovascular disease
    bio-identical progesterone and,
        80
    olive oil and, 36
    omega-3 fatty acids and, 31
    risk factors for, 21
carpet, 198
Carrot and Orange Salad, 174
carrots
    Carrot and Orange Salad, 174
    as important food to reduce
        estrogen dominance, 27,
        29–30t
    Lentil, Carrot, and Turnip Stew,
        136
    as part of diet plan, 44, 45, 48,
        53, 54, 56, 60, 61, 62, 66, 69
cauliflower
    Broccoli and Cauliflower in
        Lime Dressing, 155
    Cauliflower and Turkey Bacon
        Soup, 125
    Cauliflower Crab Cakes, 126
    as important food to reduce
        estrogen dominance, 26,
        29–30t
    Lemon-Curry Cauliflower and
        Kale, 163
    Mashed Cauliflower, 165
    as part of diet plan, 42, 43, 46,
        48, 62, 64, 69
Cauliflower and Turkey Bacon
    Soup, 125
Cauliflower Crab Cakes, 126
Celebration Salsa, 176
celery
    as important food to reduce
        estrogen dominance, 26, 27,
        29–30t
    as part of diet plan, 45, 53, 60, 66

cell growth
  bio-identical progesterone and,
    78–79
  estrogen and, 5, 21
  progesterone and, 6
cereals
  alcohol and, 41
  as important food to reduce
    estrogen dominance, 27,
    29–30t
  as part of diet plan, 44, 49, 58,
    62, 65, 70
cheese. See also dairy products
  feta (see feta)
  as part of diet plan, 44, 48, 49,
    57, 61, 62, 63, 68, 69
  Simple Cheese Toast, 187
chemicals, xenoestrogen and, 16
chicken
  Chicken and Asparagus
    Lettuce Wraps, 127
  Chicken and Cold Rice Salad,
    175
  Favorite Chicken Salad, 179
  as part of diet plan, 45, 47, 49,
    51, 52, 58, 61, 65, 66, 70, 72
  Rosemary Baked Chicken
    Breast, 143
  xenoestrogen and, 31–32
  Chicken and Asparagus
    Lettuce Wraps, 127
  Chicken and Cold Rice Salad,
    175
chickpeas
  Garlic Chickpeas and Pasta, 132
  as part of diet plan, 54, 59
  as protein source, 32t
chitosan, 95
citrus fruits. See also specific fruits
  Grilled Fish with Citrus
    Marinade, 133
  as important food to reduce
    estrogen dominance, 25
  overview of, 27, 29–30t, 37
cleaning products, 212
CME. See continuing education
coffee, 39
collard greens

as important food to reduce
    estrogen dominance, 26,
    29–30t
  as source of calcium, 35t
Colorful Turkey Casserole, 128
complete proteins, 32
compounding pharmacies
  bio-identical progesterone and,
    86
  need for, 118–20
concentration, hormone balance
    and, 15
condoms, 198
constipation, water and, 36
continuing education, marketing
    and, 77
contraception, 16, 19, 198, 199. See
    birth control pills
cooking
  cruciferous vegetables and,
    29–30t
  protein and, 32t
corn oil, avoiding, 36
cortisol, 111
cosmetics, 198, 212–13
cottage cheese. See also dairy
    products
  as part of diet plan, 42, 47, 55,
    65, 68
  Spinach Salad with Beets in
    Cottage Cheese, 188
couscous
  Cruciferous Couscous, 156
  as important food to reduce
    estrogen dominance, 27,
    29–30t
  as part of diet plan, 46, 56, 67
Cowan, Linda, 79
crab
  Cauliflower Crab Cakes, 126
  as part of diet plan, 60
cravings
  calcium-magnesium combo
    and, 92–93
  thyroid function and, 8–9
cream, bio-identical progesterone
    and, 83, 85–88, 202–5. See
    also progesterone

Creamy Coleslaw, 177
Cruciferous Couscous, 156
cruciferous vegetables
    Cruciferous Couscous, 156
    as important food to reduce
        estrogen dominance, 25
    overview of, 26, 29–30t, 37
crustaceans, chitosan and, 95
Cucumber and Yogurt Dressing,
    178
cucumbers
    Cucumber and Yogurt
        Dressing, 178
    as important food to reduce
        estrogen dominance, 27,
        29–30t
    Marinated Broccoli, Cucumber,
        and Tomato Salad, 164
    Marinated Cucumber,
        Radishes, and Onion Salad,
        184
    as part of diet plan, 44, 50, 53,
        54, 59, 60, 62, 71
cyclic hydrocarbons, 198
cyclohexane, 198

dairy products. See also specific
        products
    hormones in, 34
    as source of calcium, 35t
    xenoestrogen and, 18
dancing, 112
dehydroepiandrosterone, 93–94,
    103, 112
depression
    bio-identical progesterone and,
        83
    estrogen dominance and, 4, 14,
        17
    hormone balance and, 15
    vitamin E and, 91–92
desserts. See snacks
DHEA. See
        dehydroepiandrosterone
diagnosis, of estrogen dominance,
    19–21
diamondorganics.com, 209
diarrhea, water and, 36
diet diaries. See journaling

diet pills, need for, 4
diet plan, 41–72
digestion, water and, 36
digestive disorders, estrogen
        dominance and, 14
diindolylmethane, 90
dining out, 100
dinner. See monthly diet plan
diosgenin, 202–3
diuretics, progesterone as, 6
d-Limonene, 27
doctors
    knowledge of estrogen
        dominance and, 20–21
    marketing of hormone
        replacement and, 77
    need for, 117–18
    resources for locating, 207–8
Dr. Randolph's Natural Balance
        Cream, 202–3
Dressed-Up Asparagus, 157
dressings, salad. See under salads
drops, bio-identical progesterone
        and, 83. See also
        progesterone
dry cleaning, xenoestrogen and, 16

E1. See estrone
E2. See estradiol
E3. See estriol
Easy Pickled Beets, 158
eating. See food
education, continuing. See
        continuing education
egg, as part of diet plan, 49, 62
eggs
    Asparagus Omelet, 122
    as part of diet plan, 42, 43, 45,
        46, 47, 52, 54, 55, 59, 61, 63,
        64, 65, 67, 68, 70
    as protein source, 32t
    80-20 rule, 115–20
Eleutherococcus senticosus root, 112
elimination, water and, 36
Emerita, 204
Emory University, xx
endometriosis, 17, 21
environmental toxins. See toxins
epoxy, water bottles and, 214

erectile dysfunction, hormone
    balance and, 15
Estee Lauder, 213
esters, 198
estradiol, 26, 119–20
estriol, 26, 119–20
estrogen
    B vitamins and, 90–91
    binders of, 27
    birth control pills and, 19
    diindolylmethane and, 90
    dominance (*see* estrogen
        dominance)
    environmental, 9, 16–17, 197–99
    estrogen receptor-positive
        tumors and, 22
    food and (*see* food)
    hormone balance and, 113
    hormone replacement and (*see*
        hormone replacement)
    impact of citrus fruits on (*see*
        citrus fruits)
    impact of cruciferous
        vegetables on (*see*
        cruciferous vegetables)
    impact of insoluble fiber on (*see*
        insoluable fiber)
    impact of lignans on (*see*
        lignans)
    marketing of, 4
    phytoestrogens and, 16, 39–40
    production of "good" via food,
        26
    progesterone and, 5–6 (*see also*
        progesterone)
    thyroid hormone and, 78
    types of, 26
    vitamin E and, 91–92
    xenoestrogen and, 16–19
Estrogen, Yes or No?, 81
estrogen dominance
    cycle of, 8*f*
    example of, 11
    explanation of, 6–7
    food and (*see* food)
    hormone imbalance and, 3–5
    long-term health risks of, 21–22
    misdiagnosis of, 19–21

    self-assessment for, 12–19
    symptoms of, 14
    thyroid function and, 8–9
estrone, 26, 76, 119–20
ethanol, 198
ethers, 198
ethyl acetate, 198
ethyl ether, 198
ethyl nitrate, 198
ethylene glycol, 198
exercise. *See* physical activity

fabric softeners, 198
fast food, 100
fat
    belly (*see* belly fat)
    dehydroepiandrosterone and,
        93–94
    distribution of, 7–8
    estrogen dominance and, 7–8
    hormone balance and, 9
    meats and, 32
    oils as (*see* oils)
    saturated, 32, 38
    water and, 37
    weight control and (*see* weight
        control)
fatigue
    estrogen dominance and, 14
    hormone balance and, 15
    vitamin E and, 91–92
Favorite Chicken Salad, 179
Favorite Feta Frittata, 129–30
FDA. *See* Food and Drug
    Administration
Femhrt, 18, 75
fertilization, progesterone and, 6
feta
    Favorite Feta Frittata, 129–30
    as part of diet plan, 57, 68
    Spinach and Feta Brown Rice,
        170
fiber
    alcohol and, 41
    insoluble (*see* insoluable fiber)
    soluble (*see* soluable fiber)
fiberboard, 198
fibrocystic disease

estrogen and, 21
estrogen dominance and, 17
hormone balance and, 15
progesterone and, 6
filters
  air, 199
  water, 197
finances
  organic foods and, 209
  stress and, 103
fish
  Baked Fish with Basil, 123
  Fish New Orleans Style, 131
  Grilled Fish with Citrus
    Marinade, 133
  Grilled Salmon with Dill and
    Lemon, 134
  as important food to reduce
    estrogen dominance, 31
  Lemon Hot Fish, 135
  Not Your Ordinary Tuna Salad,
    185
  Orange-Ginger Salmon, 141
  Pan-Roasted Fish with Parsley
    and Turkey Bacon, 141
  as part of diet plan, 42, 43, 47,
    48, 50, 56, 58, 62, 64, 68, 69,
    70, 71
  as protein source, 32t
  Tuna Melt, 147
Fish New Orleans Style, 131
flaxseed
  calcium-magnesium combo
    and, 92–93
  Flaxseed and Fruit Smoothie,
    180
  as healthy oil, 36
  as important food to reduce
    estrogen dominance, 29–30t
  as part of diet plan, 42, 44, 45,
    47, 48, 49, 51, 52, 54, 55, 56,
    57, 58, 60, 61, 62, 65, 68, 69,
    70, 72
Flaxseed and Fruit Smoothie, 180
food
  daily list of, 37
  diary of, 194–96
  dining out and, 100

estrogen-increasing foods and
  (see juices)
fast food and, 100
maintenance of weight control
  and, 99–100
monthly diet plan and, 41–72
non-negotiable foods to reduce
  estrogen dominance and,
  25–30, 29–30t
other important foods to
  reduce estrogen dominance
  and, 30–37
resources for shopping for,
  208–12
Food and Drug Administration,
  21, 213
4 hydroxy pathway, 120
From Hormone Hell to Hormone
  Well, 19, 86, 215
fruits
  alcohol and, 41
  Banana in Bark, 171
  citrus (see citrus fruits)
  Flaxseed and Fruit Smoothie, 180
  overview of, 35, 37
  as part of diet plan, 45
  Yogurt and Fruit Parfait, 189
fuels, xenoestrogen and, 16
fungicides, 16

garbanzo beans. See chickpeas
garlic
  Garlic Chickpeas and Pasta, 132
  as important food to reduce
    estrogen dominance, 28
  as part of diet plan, 47, 53, 68
  Simple Greens and Garlic, 168
Garlic Chickpeas and Pasta, 132
gelcaps, bio-identical progesterone
  and, 83. See also
  progesterone
ginger
  Ginger-Lime Dressing, 181
  Orange-Ginger Salmon, 141
  as part of diet plan, 45, 57, 60,
    66
Ginger-Lime Dressing, 181
glass, 215

glues, 199
glycols, 198
goitrogens, 29–30*t*
grains, 29–30*t*. *See also* whole
    grains
grapefruit
    Grapefruit and Avocado Salad,
        182
    as important food to reduce
        estrogen dominance, 27,
        29–30*t*
    as part of diet plan, 42, 44, 46,
        47, 50, 53, 57, 63, 68, 71
Grapefruit and Avocado Salad, 182
Grated Beet Salad, 183
Green and Yellow Veggie Hash,
    159
greens
    as important food to reduce
        estrogen dominance, 26,
        29–30*t*
    Nest of Beans and Greens, 137
    as part of diet plan, 47, 53, 61,
        68
    Simple Greens and Garlic, 168
    as source of calcium, 35*t*
Grilled Asparagus with Sesame
    Seeds, 160
Grilled Fish with Citrus Marinade,
    133
Grilled Salmon with Dill and
    Lemon, 134
growth hormones, meats and,
    31–32

halogenated hydrocarbons, 198
headaches
    estrogen dominance and, 14
    hormone balance and, 15
    vitamin E and, 91–92
health, effects of hormone balance
    on, xx–xxi
The Health and Science Research
    Institute, 204
heartburn, water and, 36
herbal teas, as part of diet plan.
    See teas
herbicides, 16

herbs
    Baked Fish with Basil, 123
    Grilled Salmon with Dill and
        Lemon, 134
    Pan-Roasted Fish with Parsley
        and Turkey Bacon, 141
    as part of diet plan (*see specific
        recipes*)
    Rosemary Baked Chicken
        Breast, 143
    Rutabagas and Nutmeg, 167
herring, 31
HM Enterprises, 204
holisticphysician.com, 215
honey, as part of diet plan, 48, 54,
    60, 69
Hopkins, Virginia, 87
hormone balance
    cycle of, 8*f*
    dehydroepiandrosterone and,
        93–94
    estrogen dominance and (*see*
        estrogen)
    food and (*see* food)
    menopause and, 3
    resources for, 201–5
    stress and, 101–9
hormone level testing, resources
    for, 205–7
hormone replacement
    bio-identical (*see* bio-identical
        hormone replacement
        therapies)
    dangers of synthetic, 74–76
    marketing of, 4, 77
    menopause and, 19
    natural (*see* natural hormone
        replacement therapy)
    recent attention regarding, 74
    synthetic (*see* synthetic
        hormone replacement)
    xenoestrogen and, 18
hormonewell.com, 211, 217
hot dogs, as part of diet plan, 68
hot flashes
    bio-identical progesterone and, 83
    hormone balance and, 15
    hormone replacement and, 19

Hoy, Claire, 22
hunger, thyroid function and, 8–9
hydroxy pathways, 120
hypothalamus, bio-identical
    hormone replacement and,
    75
hypothyroidism, 8
hysterectomy, prevalence of, 13

I3C. *See* indole-3-carbinol
IACP. *See* International Academy
    of Compounding
    Pharmacists
Image Power Green Brands
    Survey, 213
incontinence, hormone balance
    and, 15
Indian-Style Brussels Sprouts, 161
indole-3-carbinol, 26, 90
industrial waste, xenoestrogen
    and, 16
infertility, estrogen dominance
    and, 17
insoluble fiber
    as important food to reduce
        estrogen dominance, 25
    overview of, 27, 29–30t, 37
insomnia. *See* sleep patterns
International Academy of
    Compounding Pharmacists,
    119, 207–8
International Cancer Journal, 76
International Society for
    Preventive Oncology, 76
International Union Against
    Cancer, 76
irritability, hormone balance and,
    15

jams, as part of diet plan, 42, 43,
    68, 71
Johns Hopkins, 79
Journal of Cell Metabolism, 31
*The Journal of the American Medical
    Association*, 76, 81
Journal of Women's Health, 82–83
journaling
    food diary and, 194–96

maintenance of weight control
    and, 101
sample of, 191–94
juices
    as option for fruit
        consumption, 29–30t
    as part of diet plan, 46, 51, 61,
        67, 72
jumping rope, 112

kale
    as important food to reduce
        estrogen dominance, 26, 29–30t
    Kale and Sauerkraut, 162
    Lemon-Curry Cauliflower and
        Kale, 163
    as part of diet plan, 50, 57, 65,
        68, 69, 71
    Spicy Kale and Beans, 145
Kale and Sauerkraut, 162
kasha, as important food to reduce
    estrogen dominance, 29–30t
ketones, 198
kidney function, water and, 37

labels
    food, 29–30t
    reading, 198
LCU. *See* life-change units
leaf lettuce, as source of calcium,
    35t
Lee, John R., 87, 206
legumes, as protein source, 32
Lemon Hot Fish, 135
Lemon-Curry Cauliflower and
    Kale, 163
lemons
    Grilled Salmon with Dill and
        Lemon, 134
    as important food to reduce
        estrogen dominance, 27, 28,
        29–30t
    Lemon Hot Fish, 135
    Lemon-Curry Cauliflower and
        Kale, 163
    as part of diet plan, 42, 43, 44,
        45, 46, 47, 48, 49, 50, 51, 52,
        53, 54, 55, 56, 57, 58, 59, 60,

lemons (cont'd)
61, 62, 63, 64, 65, 66, 67, 69,
70, 71, 72
with water, 36–37
Lentil, Carrot, and Turnip Stew, 136
lentils
as important food to reduce
estrogen dominance, 27
Lentil, Carrot, and Turnip Stew,
136
as part of diet plan, 44
as protein source, 32t
lethargy, estrogen dominance and,
13
lettuce
Chicken and Asparagus
Lettuce Wraps, 127
as part of diet plan, 47
as source of calcium, 35t
Lewis, Tene T., 101–2
libido
estrogen dominance and, 14
hormone balance and, 15
progesterone and, 6
licorice root, 112
Life Extension, 211
life-change units, stress and,
105–7, 107t
Life-flo Health Care Products, 205
lignans
estrogen and, 39
as important food to reduce
estrogen dominance, 25
overview of, 28, 29–30t, 37
lima beans, as protein source, 32t
limes
Broccoli and Cauliflower in
Lime Dressing, 155
Ginger-Lime Dressing, 181
as important food to reduce
estrogen dominance, 27,
29–30t
as part of diet plan, 45, 60, 62, 66
water and, 36
liposomal formulation, bio-
identical progesterone and,
86, 203–4
liver function, alcohol and, 39, 40

L'Oreal, 213
lunch. See monthly diet plan

magnesium, 92–93, 112
main dishes
Asparagus Omelet, 122
Baked Fish with Basil, 123
Black Beanofritos, 124
Cauliflower and Turkey Bacon
Soup, 125
Cauliflower Crab Cakes, 126
Chicken and Asparagus
Lettuce Wraps, 127
Colorful Turkey Casserole, 128
Favorite Feta Frittata, 129–30
Fish New Orleans Style, 131
Garlic Chickpeas and Pasta, 132
Grilled Fish with Citrus
Marinade, 133
Grilled Salmon with Dill and
Lemon, 134
Lemon Hot Fish, 135
Lentil, Carrot, and Turnip Stew,
136
Nest of Beans and Greens, 137
Open-Faced Veggie
Cheeseburger, 138–39
Orange-Ginger Salmon, 141
Pan-Roasted Fish with Parsley
and Turkey Bacon, 141
Quick Turkey-Stuffed Cabbage,
142
Rosemary Baked Chicken
Breast, 143
Savory Spinach and Salmon
Salad, 144
Spicy Kale and Beans, 145
Tossed Turkey Bacon and
Spinach Salad, 146
Tuna Melt, 147
Turkey, Apple, and Spinach
Pita, 149
Turkey and Asparagus Wraps, 148
Veggie Burgers, 150
mandarin oranges, as part of diet
plan, 47, 55, 68
margarine
avoiding, 36

as part of diet plan, 43, 51, 62,
    64, 68, 71, 72
Marinated Broccoli, Cucumber,
    and Tomato Salad, 164
Marinated Cucumber, Radishes,
    and Onion Salad, 184
marketing, hormone replacement
    and, 4, 77
Marketing Week, 213
Mashed Cauliflower, 165
Mayo Clinic, 82–83
meat
    alcohol and, 41
    as protein source, 32*t*
    xenoestrogen and, 16, 18, 31–32
meditation, stress and, 108–9
medmarketplace.com, 215
memory
    bio-identical progesterone and,
        82
    estrogen dominance and, 14
    hormone balance and, 15
men
    calcium and, 33
    estrogen dominance and, 9, 13–14
    supplements for (*see*
        supplements)
    symptoms of hormone
        imbalance in, 15
Menest, 18, 75
menopause
    bio-identical progesterone and,
        84
    estrogen dominance and, 13–14
    hormone imbalance and, 3
    hormone replacement and, 19
    men and (*see* andropause)
menstruation
    anovulation and, 17
    bio-identical progesterone and,
        81–82, 84
    calcium-magnesium combo
        and, 92–93
    estrogen and, 5
    estrogen dominance and, 17
    hormone balance and, 15
mental clarity, 14, 15
metabolism

dehydroepiandrosterone and,
    93–94
diindolylmethane and, 90
estrogen dominance and, 7
maintenance of weight control
    and, 99–100
progesterone and, 78
water and, 37
methanol, 198
methylethylketone, 198
microwaves, 197
migraines, estrogen dominance
    and, 14
milk, as part of diet plan, 44, 49,
    52, 58, 62, 65, 70. *See also*
    dairy products
money. *See* finances
monthly diet plan, 41–72
moods
    antidepressants and, 20
    bio-identical progesterone and,
        82
    estrogen dominance and, 17
    hormone balance and, 15
    hormone replacement and, 19
mustard greens, as important food
    to reduce estrogen
    dominance, 26, 29–30*t*
My Natural Balance Cream, 203
My Own, 217

National Institutes of Health, 76
*Natural Hormone Balance for
    Women*, 79
Natural Hormone Institute of
    America, xx
The Natural Hormone Institute of
    America, 201–2
natural hormone replacement
    therapy, 74. *See also*
    bio-identical hormone
    replacement therapies
The Natural Progesterone
    Advisory Network, 217
nervousness
    hormone balance and, 15
    vitamin E and, 91–92
Nest of Beans and Greens, 137

newsletters, 217
n-hexane, 198
night sweats
    hormone balance and, 15
    hormone replacement and, 19
NIH. *See* National Institutes of
    Health
nitrohydrocarbons, 198
Not Too Pretty: Phthalates, Beauty
    Products and the FDA, 213
Not Your Ordinary Tuna Salad,
    185
Noteloviz, Morris, 81
nuts, as protein source, 32

oat bran, as important food to
    reduce estrogen dominance,
    27
oatmeal, as important food to reduce
    estrogen dominance, 27
oils, 36, 37, 92–93. *See also* flaxseed;
    sesame seed oil
olive oil
    calcium-magnesium combo
    and, 92–93
    as healthy oil, 36
    as part of diet plan, 43, 50, 58,
    64, 68, 71
omega-3 fatty acids, 31
onions
    Marinated Cucumber,
    Radishes, and Onion Salad,
    184
    as part of diet plan, 60, 62
Open-Faced Veggie Cheeseburger,
    138–39
OPI, 213
Orange-Ginger Salmon, 141
oranges
    Beet and Orange Salad, 172
    Carrot and Orange Salad, 174
    as important food to reduce
    estrogen dominance, 27, 29–30t
    mandarin (*see* mandarin
    oranges)
    Orange-Ginger Salmon, 141
    as part of diet plan, 43, 46, 49,
    51, 54, 55, 56, 57, 59, 61, 62,

    64, 70, 72
    as source of calcium, 35t
organic cleaning products, 212
organic foods, 31–32, 198, 208–12
organicconsumer.org, 209
organicfood.com, 209
Ortho-Est, 18, 75
osteoporosis
    bio-identical progesterone and, 81
    calcium and, 33
    hormone balance and, 15
ovarian cancer, progesterone and, 6
ovaries
    anovulation and, 17
    bio-identical hormone
    replacement and, 75
    estrogen and (*see* estrogen)
    hormone balance and, 13–14
overweight, time considerations
    for, 14

P53, 79
paints, 199
Pan-Roasted Fish with Parsley and
    Turkey Bacon, 141
pantothenic acid, 112
parenting, stress and, 103
parsley root, as important food to
    reduce estrogen dominance,
    26, 29–30t
pasta
    Garlic Chickpeas and Pasta, 132
    as important food to reduce
    estrogen dominance, 29–30t
    as part of diet plan, 50, 54, 59,
    71
patenting, bio-identical hormone
    replacement therapies and,
    20–21
PCCA. *See* Professional Compounding
    Centers for America
peaches, as important food to
    reduce estrogen dominance,
    35
peanut oil, avoiding, 36
pears
    as important food to reduce
    estrogen dominance, 27, 35

as part of diet plan, 43, 47, 51,
55, 58, 63, 65
peas
as important food to reduce
estrogen dominance, 27
as source of calcium, 35*t*
pecans, as protein source, 32*t*
peptide YY, 31
perfumes, 198
pesticides, 16, 18, 198
petrochemicals, xenoestrogen and,
18
pharmaceutical hormone
replacement, 74. *See also*
hormone replacement
pharmaceutical industry
hormone replacement and, 19
marketing of hormone
replacement and, 4, 77
Prozac and, 20
recombinant bovine
somatotropin and, 34
pharmacies, compounding. *See*
compounding pharmacies
Phthalates, 213
physical activity, stress and,
111–12
physicians. *See* doctors
phytoestrogens, 16, 39–40
pills, bio-identical progesterone
and, 83. *See also*
progesterone
plant cellulose, 112
plants, phytoestrogens and, 16
plastics
water bottles and, 214–15
xenoestrogen and, 16, 18, 197
PMS. *See* premenstrual syndrome
poultry
as protein source, 32*t*
xenoestrogen and, 31–32
pregnancy, estrogen/progesterone
and, 5–6
Premarin, 18, 75–76
premature aging, hormone
balance and, 15
premenstrual syndrome
antidepressants and, 20

bio-identical progesterone and,
81–82
calcium and, 33
calcium-magnesium combo
and, 92–93
estrogen dominance and, 17
vitamin E and, 91–92
Prempro, 18, 75–76
Proctor & Gamble, 213
Products of Nature, 205
Professional Compounding
Centers for America, 119,
208
progesterone
age and, 13–14
bio-identical hormone
replacement of, 78
birth control pills and, 19
boosting levels of, 73–74
dangers of synthetic
replacement of, 74–76
estrogen and, 5–6 (*see also*
estrogen)
estrogen dominance and, 7
forms of bio-identical, 83
guidelines for use of, 84–88
health benefits of bio-identical,
78–83
maintenance of weight control
and, 99
marketing of, 77
men and, 9
resources for finding, 202–5
synthetic, 16
progestin, 16
prostate problems
cancer and, 6
hormone balance and, 15
protein, 31–32, 32*t*, 37
Prozac, 20
puberty, estrogen and, 5

pumpkin seeds
  as important food to reduce
    estrogen dominance, 29–30t
  as part of diet plan, 44, 48, 50,
    54, 65, 69, 71
PYY. *See* peptide YY

quality of life, bio-identical
    progesterone and, 82–83
Quick Turkey-Stuffed Cabbage, 142

radish
  as important food to reduce
    estrogen dominance, 26
  Marinated Cucumber,
    Radishes, and Onion Salad,
    184
  as part of diet plan, 54, 60, 62
RBA. *See* relative binding affinity
rBST. *See* recombinant bovine
    somatotropin
reading, resources for, 215–17
recombinant bovine somatotropin,
    34
red meat, 32
regulation, bio-identical
    progesterone and, 84–85
Reiss, Uzzi, 79
relationships, stress and, 103
relative binding affinity, 74, 75
relative hypothyroidism, 8
Restored Balance, Inc., 205
Revlon, 213
rice. *See* brown rice
Roasted Beets, 166
romaine lettuce, as source of
    calcium, 35t
Rosemary Baked Chicken Breast,
    143
Rush University Medical Center,
    101–2
rutabagas
  Baked Rutabaga, 152
  as important food to reduce
    estrogen dominance, 29–30t
  as part of diet plan, 45, 53, 67
  Rutabagas and Nutmeg, 167
Rutabagas and Nutmeg, 167

safecosmetics.org, 213
safflower oil, avoiding, 36
salads
  Beet and Orange Salad, 172
  Cabbage-Apple Salad, 173
  Carrot and Orange Salad, 174
  Celebration Salsa, 176
  Chicken and Cold Rice Salad, 175
  Creamy Coleslaw, 177
  Cucumber and Yogurt
    Dressing, 178
  Favorite Chicken Salad, 179
  Ginger-Lime Dressing, 181
  Grapefruit and Avocado Salad,
    182
  Grated Beet Salad, 183
  Marinated Cucumber,
    Radishes, and Onion Salad,
    184
  Not Your Ordinary Tuna Salad,
    185
  as part of diet plan, 45, 46, 49,
    51, 52, 54, 59, 61, 63, 64, 70
  Sauerkraut Salad, 186
  Savory Spinach and Salmon
    Salad, 144
  Spinach Salad with Beets in
    Cottage Cheese, 188
  Tossed Turkey Bacon and
    Spinach Salad, 146
saliva testing, 206
salmon
  alcohol and, 41
  as important food to reduce
    estrogen dominance, 31
  as part of diet plan, 43, 45, 51,
    53, 56, 59, 63, 64, 66, 72
  Savory Spinach and Salmon
    Salad, 144
  as source of calcium, 35t
saturated fat, 32, 38
sauerkraut. *See* cabbage
Sauerkraut Salad, 186
sausage, as part of diet plan, 58
Savory Spinach and Salmon Salad,
    144
schizandra berry, as adrenal
    support, 112

seeds, as important food to reduce
    estrogen dominance, 27,
    29–30t
selective serotonin reuptake
    inhibitors, 20
self-assessment, for estrogen
    dominance, 12–19
sesame seeds
    Grilled Asparagus with Sesame
        Seeds, 160
    as important food to reduce
        estrogen dominance, 28,
        29–30t
    as part of diet plan, 43, 46, 48,
        50, 53, 60, 64
    Skillet Broccoli or Asparagus
        with Sesame Seeds, 169
7-keto dehydroepiandrosterone.
    See dehydroepiandrosterone
sexual appetite. See libido
shellfish
    Cauliflower Crab Cakes, 126
    chitosan and, 95
shopping
    maintenance of weight control
        and, 99
    resources for, 208–12
side dishes. See vegetable dishes
silica, 112
Simple Cheese Toast, 187
Simple Greens and Garlic, 168
16-hydroxy pathway, 120
Skillet Broccoli or Asparagus with
    Sesame Seeds, 169
Sleep Disorders Centers of
    Southeastern Lung Care, 111
sleep patterns
    bio-identical progesterone and,
        83
    hormone replacement and, 19
    progesterone and, 6
    stress and, 110–11
    vitamin E and, 91–92
sluggishness, estrogen dominance
    and, 13
smoothies, 28, 36, 51, 56, 72, 180
snacks
    Banana in Bark, 171

Flaxseed and Fruit Smoothie,
    180
maintenance of weight control
    and, 100
Simple Cheese Toast, 187
Yogurt and Fruit Parfait, 189
sodas, 39
sodium, supplements and, 92–93
soluble fiber, 27
solvents, xenoestrogen and, 18
soup, Cauliflower and Turkey
    Bacon Soup, 125
soy products
    as bio-identical hormone
        replacement, 74
    diosgenin and, 202–3
    phytoestrogens and, 39–40
spermicides, 198
Spicy Kale and Beans, 145
spinach
    as important food to reduce
        estrogen dominance, 26, 29–30t
    as part of diet plan, 42, 43, 46,
        54, 56, 59, 61, 63, 64, 65, 68
    Savory Spinach and Salmon
        Salad, 144
    Spinach and Feta Brown Rice,
        170
    Spinach Salad with Beets in
        Cottage Cheese, 188
    Tossed Turkey Bacon and
        Spinach Salad, 146
    Turkey, Apple, and Spinach
        Pita, 149
Spinach and Feta Brown Rice, 170
Spinach Salad with Beets in
    Cottage Cheese, 188
squash
    Green and Yellow Veggie Hash,
        159
    as part of diet plan, 51, 72
    zucchini, 27, 29–30t
SSRIs. See selective serotonin
    reuptake inhibitors
stainless steel, water bottles and,
    214
stamina, hormone balance and, 15
steroids. See under adrenal function

stews, Lentil, Carrot, and Turnip
    Stew, 136
stinging nettle leaf, 112
strawberries, as important food to
    reduce estrogen dominance,
    27, 35
strength, hormone balance and, 15
stress
    inventory of, 107t
    weight control and, 101–9
sublingual drops, bio-identical
    progesterone and, 83. *See
    also* progesterone
sugar
    cravings for, 8–9
    supplements and, 92–93
sunflower oil, avoiding, 36
supplements
    adrenal function and, 112–13
    B vitamins, 90–91
    calcium, 35
    calcium D-glucarate, 89–90
    calcium-magnesium combo,
        92–93
    chitosan, 95
    dehydroepiandrosterone, 93–94
    diindolylmethane, 90
    hormone support and, xix
    resources for brands of, 210–11
    vitamin E, 91–92
suppositories, bio-identical
    progesterone and, 83. *See
    also* progesterone
swimming, 112
synthetic hormone replacement,
    74, 199. *See also* hormone
    replacement

tahini, as important food to reduce
    estrogen dominance, 28,
    29–30t
tangelos, as important food to
    reduce estrogen dominance,
    27, 29–30t
tangerines
    as important food to reduce
        estrogen dominance, 27,
        29–30t

as part of diet plan, 49, 56, 62,
    64, 70
tearfulness, hormone balance and,
    15
teas
    caffeine and, 39
    as part of diet plan (*see*
        monthly diet plan)
television, maintenance of weight
    control and, 100
testes, bio-identical hormone
    replacement and, 75
testicular tissue, progesterone and,
    9
testosterone
    dehydroepiandrosterone and,
        93–94
    diindolylmethane and, 90
    hormone balance and, 113
    as sex hormone, 5
themonspa.com, 213
thinking difficulties. *See* mental
    clarity
thyroid function
    cruciferous vegetables and,
        29–30t
    estrogen and, 78
    estrogen dominance and, 8–9
    phytoestrogens and, 40
tomatoes
    as important food to reduce
        estrogen dominance, 27,
        29–30t
    Marinated Broccoli, Cucumber,
        and Tomato Salad, 164
    as part of diet plan, 44, 46, 50,
        58, 68, 71
tortillas, as part of diet plan, 60
Tossed Turkey Bacon and Spinach
    Salad, 146
toxins
    estrogen dominance and, 16–17
    hormone balance and, 9
    reduction of, 197–99
trichloroethylene, 198
tri-est, 119–20
trimethylglycine, 112
trout, 31

*The Truth About the Drug
Companies*, 77
tuna
as important food to reduce
estrogen dominance, 31
Not Your Ordinary Tuna Salad,
185
as part of diet plan, 46, 55, 67
Tuna Melt, 147
Tuna Melt, 147
turkey
Cauliflower and Turkey Bacon
Soup, 125
Colorful Turkey Casserole, 128
Pan-Roasted Fish with Parsley
and Turkey Bacon, 141
as part of diet plan, 44, 46, 48,
49, 53, 54, 55, 56, 58, 60, 61,
63, 65, 67, 68, 69, 71
Quick Turkey-Stuffed Cabbage,
142
Tossed Turkey Bacon and
Spinach Salad, 146
Turkey, Apple, and Spinach
Pita, 149
Turkey and Asparagus Wraps,
148
xenoestrogen and, 31–32
Turkey, Apple, and Spinach Pita,
149
Turkey and Asparagus Wraps, 148
turnip
as important food to reduce
estrogen dominance, 26,
29–30*t*
Lentil, Carrot, and Turnip Stew,
136
as part of diet plan, 44
2-hydroxy pathway, 120

Unilever, 213
University of Missouri, 214
urinary difficulties, hormone
balance and, 15
uterine cancer, progesterone and, 6
uterine function,
estrogen/progesterone and,
5–6

vaginal dryness, hormone balance
and, 15
vaginal gels, 198
vegetable dishes
Asian Cabbage, 151
Baked Rutabaga, 152
Beets and Brussels Sprouts, 153
Best Baked Beans, 154
Broccoli and Cauliflower in
Lime Dressing, 155
Cruciferous Couscous, 156
Dressed-Up Asparagus, 157
Easy Pickled Beets, 158
Green and Yellow Veggie Hash,
159
Grilled Asparagus with Sesame
Seeds, 160
Indian-Style Brussels Sprouts,
161
Kale and Sauerkraut, 162
Lemon-Curry Cauliflower and
Kale, 163
Marinated Broccoli, Cucumber,
and Tomato Salad, 164
Mashed Cauliflower, 165
Roasted Beets, 166
Rutabagas and Nutmeg, 167
Simple Greens and Garlic, 168
Skillet Broccoli or Asparagus
with Sesame Seeds, 169
Spinach and Feta Brown Rice,
170
vegetable stearate, 112
vegetables
cruciferous (*see* cruciferous
vegetables)
washing, 198
veggie burgers
Open-Faced Veggie
Cheeseburger, 138–39
as part of diet plan, 45, 51, 62,
66, 72
as protein source, 32*t*
recipe for, 150

Virginia Hopkin's Healthwatch, 217
visualization, stress and, 109
vitamin C, 112
vitamin E, 91–92
vitamins. *See specific vitamin name*; supplements

walking, 112
walnuts, as protein source, 32*t*
water
  bottles and, 214–15
  filtering, 197
  importance of, 36–37
water retention, hormone balance and, 15
weight control
  B vitamins and, 90–91
chitosan and, 95
  cycle of gain and, 8*f*
  estrogen dominance and, 4, 7–8, 14, 17
  hormone balance and, 15
  maintenance of, 99–101
  stress and, 101–9
What Your Doctor May Not Tell You About Breast Cancer, 206
What Your Doctor May Not Tell You About Menopause, 87
wheat
  as important food to reduce estrogen dominance, 27, 29–30*t*
  as part of diet plan, 42, 43, 44, 47, 50, 51, 53, 54, 55, 59, 60, 63, 64, 65, 68, 71, 72
wheat bran
  as important food to reduce estrogen dominance, 27, 29–30*t*
  as part of diet plan, 44, 49, 58, 62, 65, 70
Whole Foods Market, 208–9
whole grains
  alcohol and, 41

as important food to reduce estrogen dominance, 27, 29–30*t*
  as part of diet plan, 42, 43, 44, 47, 49, 50, 51, 53, 55, 58, 59, 60, 62, 63, 64, 65, 68, 70, 71, 72
  resources for, 211–12
"Why Drinking Water Really Is the Key to Weight Loss", 37
Wild Oats, 209
wild yams
  as adrenal support, 112
  as bio-identical hormone replacement, 74, 85
  diosgenin and, 202–3
women
  calcium and, 33
  estrogen dominance and, 12–13
  supplements for (*see* supplements)
  symptoms of hormone imbalance in, 15
Women in Balance, 217

xenoestrogen, 16–19, 31–32, 197, 212

yams, wild. *See* wild yams
yoga, 112
yogurt
  Cucumber and Yogurt Dressing, 178
  flaxseed oil and, 36
  lignans and, 28
  as part of diet plan, 42, 45, 48, 51, 52, 53, 54, 57, 59, 60, 61, 66, 69, 72
  as source of calcium, 35*t*
  Yogurt and Fruit Parfait, 189
Yogurt and Fruit Parfait, 189

Zava, David, 206
ZRT Laboratories, 207
zucchini, 27, 29–30*t*